Objective Structured Clinical Examination
for Psychiatric Trainees

Objective Structured Clinical Examination for Psychiatric Trainees

Jaap van der Boom, Joseph Tony, Srinivasa Thirumalai

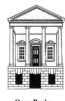

Quay Books
MA Healthcare Limited

Quay Books Division, MA Healthcare Limited, Jesses Farm, Snow Hill, Dinton, Salisbury, Wiltshire, SP3 5HN

British Library Cataloguing-in-Publication Data
A catalogue record is available for this book

© MA Healthcare Limited 2003
ISBN 1 85642 271 2

Printed in the UK by Cromwell Press, Trowbridge

To our families

Contents

Foreword   ix

Introduction   xi

Section one: History-taking skills

1.	Obsessive compulsive behaviour	3,	6,	11
2.	Telephone advice about a confused patient	3,	6,	12
3.	A reclusive patient	3,	6,	13
4.	Delusions and formal thought disorder	3,	7,	14
5.	Opiate dependence	4,	7,	16
6.	Post-traumatic stress disorder	4,	8,	18
7.	Alcohol dependence	4,	8,	19
8.	Depression/biological symptoms	4,	8,	20
9.	Psychosexual history	4,	9,	22
10.	Anxiety	5,	9,	25
11.	Lack of energy and paranoia	5,	9,	26
12.	Sleeping difficulties	5,	10,	27
13.	Grief	5,	10,	28

Section two: Examination skills

14.	Frontal lobe function	33,	36,	40
15.	Capacity to refuse consent to treatment	33,	36,	41
16.	Risk assessment of a suicidal patient	33,	36,	43
17.	Assessment for akathisia	33,	37,	44
18.	Insight/attitude	34,	37,	46
19.	Eating disorder	34,	37,	49
20.	Thyroid	34,	37,	51
21.	First rank symptoms	34,	38,	52
22.	Suicidal intent after an overdose	34,	38,	54
23.	Personality	35,	38,	56
24.	Mini Mental State Examination	35,	39,	58

Section three: Procedure skills

25.	Testing of arm and hand function	63,	65,	67
26.	Obtain consent and perform an ECG recording	63,	65,	68
27.	Alcohol dependence — physical examination	63,	65,	69
28.	Opiate dependence — physical examination	63,	65,	71

29. Extra-pyramidal side-effects — physical examination   63,   65,   73
30. Neuroleptic malignant syndrome   64,   66,   74
31. Serotonin syndrome   64,   66,   76
32. Examination of cranial nerves (1)   64,   66,   77
33. Examination of cranial nerves (2)   64,   66,   79
34. Fundoscopic examination of the eye   64,   66,   80

Section four: Communication skills

35. Discuss laboratory results   85,   88,   91
36. Drug misuse in pregnancy   85,   88,   92
37. Information for out-patient ECT   85,   88,   94
38. Prognosis in schizophrenia   86,   88,   95
39. Aetiology of a psychotic episode   86,   89,   96
40. Starting a patient on clozapine   86,   89,   98
41. Clozapine reaction   86,   89,   100
42. Alzheimer's disease   87,   89,   101
43. Dementia treatment   87,   90,   103
44. Starting a patient on lithium   87,   90,   105
45. Discussing ECT as a treatment option   87,   90,   106

Useful resources   109

Foreword

In this book, three psychiatrists acutely familiar with MRCPsych have taken the groundbreaking step of laying out advice on technique and factual examples of Objective Structured Clinical Examinations (OSCEs). OSCEs are, I feel, a fairer and more stimulating exam than the single case predecessor.

Reading this book is interesting, informative and thought-provoking. As well as for candidates I commend it to tutors and trainers as a tool for sharpening up structured thinking and informing approaches to OSCE teaching.

For candidates, good preparation must go beyond this book into wide reading, extensive and thorough history taking in your clinical placements and the assimilation of a very broad factual knowledge overlapping with multiple choice preparation from the syllabus. The many potential areas of structured facts lend themselves well to your own encyclopaedic notes, posters blue-tacked on the back of the lavatory door and making your own audio cassette tapes for revision during motoring.

Smile at the examiners confidently (not, of course, sycophantically) and enjoy acting the part of a competent psychiatrist. Remember that the best antidote to performance anxiety is performance enthusiasm. Good luck and do lots of work.

Professor Stephen Martin
Consultant Neuropsychiatrist
Westminster Health Care Group
October 2003

Introduction

This book is intended for those trainees preparing for the MRCPsych Part 1 examination. Objective structured clinical examinations (OSCEs) are being used to test a broad range of subjects and skills in a quantifiable and valid form.

The OSCE format was first used in the spring of 2003.

An OSCE differs from the traditional 'long case' exam, by using simulated cases or patients. The aim of this design is to reduce the likelihood of candidates having varying experiences with the same patient. OSCEs are designed to ensure that a range of skills are tested, with scores being allocated against clear and explicit criteria. They are more objective because each candidate is observed and assessed in a similar situation.

In the OSCEs, the roles are played by actors or in certain stations an anatomical model will be used. In that way a wide range of skills can be tested without having to recruit actual patients with specific symptoms or illnesses. Anatomical models allow skills to be tested that would normally be difficult to conduct on actors or volunteers, eg. cardio-pulmonary resuscitation.

Candidates usually rotate around twelve OSCE stations, which last for seven minutes. The candidates all start at a different station and then rotate, completing the remaining stations. A bell is rung forty seconds before the seven minutes are over. There may be one rest station.

Each OSCE station is designed to assess a particular skill within the core curriculum. The list of skills to be tested includes:

- eliciting a relevant history
- making a diagnosis
- clinical examination
- discussion of treatment options
- obtaining consent for treatment or procedures
- performing specific procedures
- discussion of test results and prognosis
- prescribing appropriate treatment.

How to use this book

This book contains a series of OSCE examples. The main sections divide the OSCEs into those that focus on history-taking, communication, procedural and specific examination skills. Within each section are instructions for candidates, actors and examiners. The instructions for examiners include marking criteria and sample answers. The answers that we have written are only a rough guide as to what you might say or do in the actual exam. With practice, you will hopefully be able to improve on our answers and develop your own personal style, with which you feel comfortable.

We would suggest that if possible you try to practice by doing role play in a small group. One person could take the role of the candidate, another could be the actor and the others could act as examiners. It is also important that somebody keeps a track of the time. Try to stick to the time frame of seven minutes and the warning with forty seconds to go, so that you get a feel for it. Candidates are given a minute to read the instructions and gather their thoughts. The actors may need some more time to get into their role.

For the role of examiner we have given some suggestions about the way the OSCEs can be approached. This is, however, not the only correct way. It is important you come up with an approach that shows understanding and insight. We have also added some ratings which can be used by the examiners. We would suggest you go over the OSCE afterwards, to see in which areas you have done well and where you could still improve. You will benefit most from these sessions when you use positive feedback.

If you can, get an SpR or a consultant involved.

For the 'Procedural' OSCEs we have provided relevant check lists as physical examination does not easily lend itself to being assessed in a textbook. 'Procedural' OSCEs might also be best done in groups.

How are OSCEs marked?

Table Introduction.1 shows a specimen check-list for an OSCE station. You will notice the different and very specific attributes of a candidate that are examined.

Table Introduction.1: Check-list for an OSCE station

	Excellent A	Good B	Average C	Fail D	Severe fail E
Introduction					
Rapport					
Consent					
Listening skills					
Verbal					
facilitation					
Question framing					
Emotional content					
Explanation					
Diagnostic					
criteria					
Factual					
knowledge					
Summarization					
Patient's concerns					
and perceptions					
Ending					

Preparing for the examination

⌘ It is useful, and makes sense to practice OSCEs in groups.

⌘ Make a list of likely OSCEs, dividing them according to skills tested or even disorders.

⌘ Ask for practice sessions with local SpRs or consultant trainers, who have an interest in the field.

⌘ Practice often, though how often is up to you! We have found that it is useful to repeat OSCEs after an interval of up to several days, to see whether there is an actual improvement in your scores.

⌘ Practice all the roles so that you not only get to know what it is like on the 'other' side, but also get an idea as to what really works or impresses.

⌘ Try to stick to exam conditions — the pressure can be intense!

Tips for success on the day

⌘ Arrive early and look your best.

⌘ Introduce yourself to the patient and outline what you are going to do in broad terms.

⌘ Listen to the patient. You might have a task to do, but you are also being observed on the details of your interaction with the patient.

⌘ Pick up clues in what the patient says to you. They might give you openings or ways out of difficult situations.

⌘ Adapt to the situation. Although we have tried to cover as many potential areas as we could, be prepared for anything.

⌘ Stop yourself from asking questions as if from a list. Practice different types of questions including open-ended questions ('Tell me about...') that allow the patient to expand on his/her answers.

⌘ Be sensitive to the situation and the patient.

⌘ Obtain consent for any procedure.

⌘ Explain everything!

⌘ Watch your technique — don't be careless in disposing of used medical instruments.

Remember that there are many stations: you have more than one opportunity to show that you measure up to the standard. Even if you remember a vital point/question some way into the question, try to incorporate it into what you are doing. You cannot be failed for correcting a mistake.

What are the examiners looking for?

⌘ Confidence.

⌘ Good communication.

⌘ Flexibility in questioning style.

⌘ Reasonable factual knowledge.

⌘ Competence in performing procedures.
⌘ A balanced approach.
⌘ Empathy.
⌘ Treating the station as if it were 'real' life.
⌘ Sensitivity to a patient's distress or anxiety.
⌘ A demonstration of reasonable control of interview.

We hope that by using these OSCEs to revise your skills, you will be better prepared to face the actual examination. Good Luck!

Jaap van der Boom
Joseph Tony
Srinivasa Thirumalai

September 2003

Section one:
History-taking skills

Instructions for candidates

1. Obsessive compulsive behaviour

A twenty-seven-year-old single woman, who works as a dental assistant, has come to see you. She lives with her elderly parents. She is very troubled by thoughts about pushing somebody into the road, in front of oncoming traffic. She has been resisting these impulses but has become increasingly anxious.

Assess her symptoms.

2. Telephone advice about a confused patient

You are the senior house officer on call and will be asked for some advice by the surgical house officer.

3. A reclusive patient

A twenty-nine-year-old man has been referred to you by his general practitioner (GP). His parents have been complaining that he just sits in his room and is reluctant to leave the house. He has never had a partner and has not made any effort to find work since he lost his job at a printing company eight years ago.

Assess his symptoms.

4. Delusions and formal thought disorder

A young man has been admitted to your ward. Nursing staff tell you that it is difficult to understand what he is saying.

Interview him and establish the content and conviction of his beliefs and whether or not he exhibits formal thought disorder.

5. Opiate dependence

You are asked to see a twenty-one-year-old man at your outpatient clinic. This man has a history of heroin use.

Take a history and screen for opiate dependence.

6. Post-traumatic stress disorder

This forty-four-year-old man was involved in a train accident about four months ago. He escaped death after being trapped in the train wreckage for four hours. Since then, he has suffered from several problems including irritability, feeling emotionally numb, and avoiding travel on trains. His GP feels that he may have post-traumatic stress disorder.

Elicit relevant history and confirm the provisional diagnosis.

7. Alcohol dependence

This thirty-year-old man drinks alcohol on a daily basis.

Elicit relevant history to decide whether he is alcohol-dependent.

8. Depression/biological symptoms

This sixty-eight-year-old man has attended the A&E department complaining of chest pain. The casualty medical officer (CMO) has investigated him fully and has found no evidence of cardiac problems. However, the patient has not been sleeping well and has lost weight since his wife was diagnosed with breast cancer three months ago. The CMO thinks this patient might be depressed.

Clarify the presenting complaints and assess for biological symptoms of depression.

9. Psychosexual history

Your first patient in the psychiatric out-patient clinic is a thirty-two-year-old man, who had been to his GP complaining of relationship dificulties. His partner left him two weeks earlier.

Ascertain his psychosexual history.

10. Anxiety

You have been asked to see this twenty-seven-year-old housewife by the medical senior house officer. She has presented herself to the local A&E department with acute chest pain, but no organic cause has been found. This is her third presentation in two days.

Assess her presentation, focusing on her anxiety symptoms.

11. Lack of energy and paranoia

You have been asked to see this twenty-year-old man, who complains of a lack of energy and feeling that people are looking at him in the street. He used to live with his parents, but has recently moved out. He worked in a supermarket after dropping out of college, but gave this up a while ago.

Assess his presenting complaints.

12. Sleeping difficulties

This twenty-six-year-old woman has been referred to you because she has difficulty sleeping at night.

Assess her presenting complaints and give her advice for her sleep problem.

13. Grief

You have been asked to see this sixty-nine-year-old man by his GP. His wife died unexpectedly six months ago. He has two daughters, who have been trying to support him, but he has found it very difficult to cope on his own and has been neglecting himself. His daughters have expressed increasing concern about his well-being.

Instructions for actors

1. Obsessive compulsive behaviour

You are a twenty-seven-year-old single lady, who lives with her elderly parents and works as a dental assistant. You have had frequent intrusive thoughts since witnessing an elderly woman being nearly hit by a car, several years ago. The thoughts are about pushing people into the road, especially elderly, frail people and children who are standing at the roadside. You also feel the urge to push elderly people over when you walk past them. You recognize these thoughts as your own, but try to resist them strongly.

You take a long time to get ready to go out in the morning. You have to follow a rigid routine with your bathing and dressing. If you don't follow the routine exactly, you have to begin it all over again. At work you have to check repeatedly whether you supplied the dentist with the right materials and spend a lot of time cleaning the dental equipment.

You want to know whether anything can help you get rid of your problems.

2. Telephone advice about a confused patient

The conversation takes place over the phone.

You are a surgical house officer, who has been asked to see a fifty-six-year-old man, on the orthopaedic ward. He fractured his ankle the day before and underwent internal fixation. He cannot weight-bear. This evening he has become very confused, has started shaking and is very anxious. You are unsure as to how to handle the situation and have decided to phone the psychiatric SHO for advice. You are very worried and explain that the patient has gone completely berserk. You think he has become 'schizophrenic' and ask for urgent help.

When prompted, you look in the notes and find that the patient apparently is a heavy drinker, who has been having up to eight pints of lager a day, and seems not to have had any alcohol since admission.

At some point during this conversation you will ask whether you can give the patient some Haloperidol.

3. A reclusive patient

You are a twenty-nine-year-old single man. You have been referred to the psychiatrist after your parents complained to your GP that you never leave the house. You cover the lower part of your face with a scarf and your hand. Initially, you are vague about your reasons for staying indoors. You 'just don't feel like going out'. You spend most of your time watching TV and playing computer games.

When prompted, you explain that you are unhappy about your chin. You think it is far too big and believe it makes you repulsive.

You became increasingly preoccupied with your appearance about twelve years ago when you were passing through puberty. You studied yourself in the mirror repeatedly and felt that people were staring at you in the street. You became withdrawn and eventually lost your part-time job because of absenteeism. You have been reluctant to go out to work since. You have never had a partner and believe that nobody would be attracted to you because of your looks. You often feel low and have had suicidal thoughts on and off, but have never tried to end your life. You do not hold any other unusual beliefs.

4. Delusions and formal thought disorder

You are twenty-one years old. Prior to this admission, you have never been in a psychiatric hospital. Your thoughts are muddled. When asked a question, you talk around the topic for a while before returning to the original question, which you then answer. You are convinced that MI5, the Government's Secret Service is looking for you in connection with Princess Diana's death. You don't know how you arrived at this conclusion. You are sure that people are watching you and listening in to your every conversation. You get special messages from the radio and television. You are unable to explain how these things are happening. You are fully convinced of these beliefs. You have observed how the chairs have been arranged in this room and you are convinced that 'they' are nearby.

5. Opiate dependence

You are a twenty-one-year-old man, who regularly uses heroin (which you call 'gear'). You mostly inject the heroin but also snort it up to three or four times a day. You also snort cocaine occasionally. On average, you spend about seventy to one hundred pounds a day on drugs. Occasionally, you inject yourself with a cocktail of up to three or four drugs. You have been using illicit drugs regularly for the last three years, after your release from prison. In that time, you have come to need more and more heroin to get the same pleasurable effect. When you have been off the heroin for longer than a few hours, you suffer from stomach cramps, muscle cramps, goose flesh, a runny nose, and yawn excessively. You spend most of your waking hours either taking the drugs or looking for money for them. Three months ago, you were taken to the local A&E department after accidentally overdosing on a cocktail of drugs. You have had two previous overdoses and had to spend four nights in the intensive care unit on one occasion. You have never attended appointments at the local drugs service, and have never seen a psychiatrist. You do not share needles or any injecting equipment (which you call your 'works'). You were told by your former GP that you had Hepatitis B and C about one year ago, but refused to visit the local GUM clinic for appropriate treatment. In the past, your urine has tested positive for heroin, cocaine and methadone on more than three visits to your GP. Your habit is funded by shoplifting and burglary. You are keen to give up drugs and have moved house to start a new life. You want to be realistic with your intentions and have come to ask to be started on methadone.

6. Post-traumatic stress disorder

You are a forty-four-year-old man, with no previous history of mental illness. You have been commuting by train to work in central London for the last ten years. Two months ago your train was involved in a serious crash. You lost a close friend and were yourself trapped in the wreckage for four hours before you were rescued. A child sitting near you had to have a leg amputated. Another friend who was involved in the same incident has been told that he has severe post-traumatic stress, and has been referred by his GP for counselling.

Since the accident, you have had to resign from work as you cannot bring yourself to travel by train, let alone go near a station. Your mood has been low, and your wife has commented on your irritability. You are troubled by flashbacks of the accident, which happen several times a day, and your sleep is disrupted by recurrent nightmares on similar themes.

You have lost interest in playing golf, have not been meeting with your friends and find it difficult to be around your family, who do not appreciate what you are going through. Everything seems to be an effort. The relationship with your wife has deteriorated and you are now desperate for help.

7. Alcohol dependence

You are a thirty-year-old man, who lives away from his girlfriend and two-year-old daughter. For the past six months, you have been drinking wine or beer on a daily basis. Recently, you have noticed that you wake up tremulous and sweaty in the mornings, and this is only relieved with a quick drink. Once you have started though, you cannot stop, and so continue to drink all day. You now drink only whiskey, and need at least a bottle a day just to feel 'normal.' You have not been able to stop, and whenever you go out, are constantly craving a drink. You only want help because your girlfriend is threatening to leave you.

8. Depression/biological symptoms

You are a sixty-eight-year-old man, whose wife was diagnosed with breast cancer three months ago. Since then, your mood has been low, you have lost interest in gardening and you feel tired all the time. You wake up at 4.00 am every morning and cannot get back to sleep. Your appetite is poor and you have lost two stone in weight. You cannot concentrate on the crossword or read the newspaper. You also have high blood pressure and have recently started taking a new medication for this. Today, you went to the A&E department because you had fleeting chest pains and thought you were having a heart attack. Now the casualty doctor wants you to see a psychiatrist.

9. Psychosexual history

You are a thirty-two-year-old man, who has come to a psychiatric out-patient clinic. Your GP, who saw you three days, earlier referred you there. You had complained of difficulties in your relationships. Your boyfriend, who left you two weeks ago, had phoned to say that he had been to the GUM clinic for Hepatitis and HIV tests. You panicked and started worrying that you might have contracted a sinister infection from him or other previous partners, with whom you have had unprotected sex.

10. Anxiety

You are a twenty-seven-year-old housewife with two young children. Lately, there have been rows with your husband because of financial problems. Your father, with whom you were very close, passed away last year. You have been rather worried about your health, but do not feel particularly depressed.

For the last six months you have been having frequent chest pains. During an episode, which can last up to an hour in total, you are short of breath, and have palpitations and a feeling of tightness across your chest. Your mouth and fingertips tingle. You feel restless and worry that you are having a heart attack. You are not sure why it happens, but when you worry about getting another attack it tends to be worse. These episodes have been getting more frequent and now occur at least a few times a day. You decided to go to A&E today, your third visit in two days, because the episodes have not resolved.

11. Lack of energy and paranoia

You are a twenty-year-old man who feels tired all the time. Since your teens you have felt as if people have been talking about you in the street. You dropped out of an art course at college, and worked for a few months in a supermarket. You lost your job for being off sick too often, alhough it was really because you were not motivated to go to work at all. Your parents have given up on you and you now live alone in a council flat, claiming social security benefits. When asked about your alcohol and drug intake, you mention that you like to smoke the odd 'joint.'

You then admit to smoking up to five a day, and the habit costs you about £30 a week. You do not think that it harms you in any way, and, anyway, it has now been made fully legal by the Government.

12. Sleeping difficulties

You are a twenty-six-year-old woman, who lives alone and works in a radio station. You have found it difficult to sleep for many months now.

Your last meal of the day is at around 9.00 pm. You avoid tea and coffee. Your flat overlooks a busy road and traffic sounds keep you awake for the next two hours. You usually go to bed at around 11.00 pm and watch television for an hour before you switch off the light and try to sleep. Lately, you have been tossing and turning in bed for a few hours more. You try to distract your mind by watching more television and having a cola drink, before you are finally able to get to sleep at around 3.00 or 4.00 am. You struggle to wake up the next morning in time for your day's work.

You mention that you used Diazepam for a while, which seemed to help. Your GP decided, however, that she could not continue to prescribe it. You want to know whether you can have some more Diazepam.

13. Grief

You are a sixty-nine-year old widower, who used to work at a bank. Your wife died unexpectedly six months ago. You were married for almost forty years. She used to be forceful woman, who took most of the decisions in your marriage. She had a range of hobbies and an active social life. You are a rather withdrawn man and mostly preferred to stay at home. You often felt belittled by her but find it hard to admit this. She died at the age of sixty-three of a massive stroke, while away at a church meeting. You were at home and were told several minutes later that she had been taken to hospital in an ambulance. By the time you made it there, she had already passed on.

Your two daughters were in charge at the funeral, and you were in the background.

Your daughters are both married and live some distance away. They have been trying to support you after your wife's death, but are both working and have busy family lives.

For some time afterwards, you felt numb inside. Then, you found yourself increasingly weepy. Now, you cannot settle in bed and often wake up in the middle of the night. You do not feel like eating and have lost about half a stone in weight. You often feel as if it was all a dream and that your wife will be coming home in a little while. Sometimes, you think that you can hear her opening the door. You feel tired all the time and have no interest in caring for yourself. You are still angry with her friends from church because they failed to call you straight away after she collapsed.

You are finding it very hard to come to terms with your loss and would like to know whether anything can be done about it.

Instructions for examiners

1. Obsessive compulsive behaviour

Introduces him/herself.
Shows empathy and respect.
Asks open and closed questions.

Introduction | A | | B | | C | | D | | E | |

Question framing | A | | B | | C | | D | | E | |

Verbal facilitation | A | | B | | C | | D | | E | |

⌘ Explores symptom history, precipitating factors and associated problems:

> *Can you tell me something more about the thoughts you have been having?*
> *How often do you have these thoughts?*
> *What do you do when you get these thoughts?*
> *Where do they come from?*
> *Is there anything you try to do to stop these thoughts?*
> *Do you try to resist or suppress these thoughts?*

Checks obsessional symptoms | A | | B | | C | | D | | E | |

⌘ Explores what she does in order to neutralize these thoughts:

> *Do you use mental acts like praying, counting or saying words quietly?*
> *Do you wash or clean things a lot?*
> *Do you check things?*
> *Are you concerned about orderliness or symmetry?*
> *Do you find that your daily routines take up a lot of time?*

Checks compulsive symptoms | A | | B | | C | | D | | E | |

⌘ Asks about associated symptoms, such as:

- general anxiety
- panic attacks
- depression
- phobia.

Associated symptoms |A| |B| |C| |D| |E| |

Mentions behaviour therapy, CBT and medication, in particular SSRI antidepressants.

Discusses therapy |A| |B| |C| |D| |E| |

Addresses patient's concerns |A| |B| |C| |D| |E| |

Global rating |A| |B| |C| |D| |E| |

2. Telephone advice about a confused patient

Answers the phone call.
Is polite, pleasant and helpful.

Communication |A| |B| |C| |D| |E| |

Explanation |A| |B| |C| |D| |E| |

⌘ Explores the present situation and information about the patient, including:

- background information, like marital status, work etc.
- circumstances of the injury and admission
- past psychiatric history
- alcohol or drug dependence
- physical condition
- medication.

History taking |A| |B| |C| |D| |E| |

Explores organic causes |A| |B| |C| |D| |E| |

⌘ Explore:

- alcohol intake and degree of dependence
- physical withdrawal symptoms
- symptoms of delirium tremens
- neurological symptoms
- management until now.

Checks alcohol history |A| |B| |C| |D| |E| |

⌘ Gives advice about:

- safe environment, appropriate staffing, help with orientation

- detoxification regime with chlordiazepoxide (Librium) in a reducing dose, starting with at least 20 mg qds
- alternative — other short acting benzodiazepine
- prescribing an anti-emetic
- avoiding haloperidol
- risk of withdrawal seizures
- risk of Wernicke's encephalopathy
- prophylaxis with thiamine supplementation or multivitamins (pabrinex) (multivitamins best given i.v. because of poor oral absorption).

Offer to see patient yourself if necessary.

Management
$\boxed{\text{A}\quad\text{B}\quad\text{C}\quad\text{D}\quad\text{E}}$

Global rating
$\boxed{\text{A}\quad\text{B}\quad\text{C}\quad\text{D}\quad\text{E}}$

3. A reclusive patient

Is friendly and establishes rapport.
Explains the reason for the assessment.
Starts with asking open questions.
Asks questions with sensitivity.

Introduction
$\boxed{\text{A}\quad\text{B}\quad\text{C}\quad\text{D}\quad\text{E}}$

Communication
$\boxed{\text{A}\quad\text{B}\quad\text{C}\quad\text{D}\quad\text{E}}$

Verbal facilitation
$\boxed{\text{A}\quad\text{B}\quad\text{C}\quad\text{D}\quad\text{E}}$

⌘ Explores reasons why he does not leave the house, for example:

- social phobia
- other phobias
- depression
- delusional beliefs
- negative symptoms
- body dysmorphic disorder.

Identification of presenting complaint
$\boxed{\text{A}\quad\text{B}\quad\text{C}\quad\text{D}\quad\text{E}}$

⌘ Explores:

- duration of this belief
- intensity with which held
- precipitating factors
- evidence.

Exploration of complaint | A | B | C | D | E |

⌘ Explores:

- low mood
- psychotic symptoms
- risk of deliberate self-harm (DSH).

Issues of risk | A | B | C | D | E |

⌘ Concludes and makes suggestions for further treatment, such as:

- Cognitive behaviour therapy (CBT)
- Selective serotonin reuptake inhibitors (SSRIs)
- clomipramine.

Discusses treatment | A | B | C | D | E |

Global rating | A | B | C | D | E |

4. Delusions and formal thought disorder

Establishes good rapport.
Allows patient to speak.
Briefly enquires about patient's stay in hospital.
Asks open-ended questions.
Does not directly confront patient's beliefs.
Shows empathy and demonstrates understanding of situation.

Introduction | A | B | C | D | E |

Communication | A | B | C | D | E |

Listening skills | A | B | C | D | E |

Question framing/verbal facilitation | A | B | C | D | E |

Use of language | A | B | C | D | E |

⌘ Checks thought process:

Do you feel that your thoughts get mixed up or that you can't think as clearly as before? Do you feel that you are unable to focus your thoughts? Is there anything wrong with how you've been thinking lately? Are you finding it hard to express yourself?

⌘ Checks for delusional thoughts:

Paranoia

Do you feel people are out to harm you?
Do you think they will harm you?
Are they speaking about you behind your back?

Persecution

Do you feel that specific people or agents are trying to harm you in any way?
Are they trying to conspire against you?
Do you feel that you are under observation? Are people watching you or listening to you? Are they using special equipment?

Reference and misinterpretation

Do you feel people say or do things that convey a special meaning to you?
Are people discussing you or gossiping about you all the time? How do they do this?
Do you receive any messages from the television or radio? Have you seen or read anything with special meaning for you?
Do you get special meanings from the way things are placed or arranged?

Delusion of grandiose ability/identity

Do you have special powers or abilities?
Are you someone special? Have you been selected for a special task or purpose?
Do you belong to royalty or are your family different from others in any special way?

History |A| |B| |C| |D| |E| |

⌘ Checks for other delusions such as delusions of guilt, responsibility, poverty, religious or alien identity, and paranormal phenomena or abilities.

⌘ Establishes whether these are primary or secondary delusions.

Checks definition |A| |B| |C| |D| |E| |

⌘ Establishes whether these are partial or complete delusions. This means establishing the degree of conviction in the beliefs.

Checks fixity of beliefs |A| |B| |C| |D| |E| |

⌘ Establishes the amount of systematization of the belief system. Also assesses the degree of evasiveness in answering questions, the level of preoccupation with these beliefs and the extent to which the patient has acted on these beliefs.

Looks for evasiveness, systematisation, acting out, and coping strategies

| A | B | C | D | E |

Global rating

| A | B | C | D | E |

5. Opiate dependence

Introduces himself/herself.
Explains the purpose of the interview.
Develops rapport.
Empathises with the patient.
Demonstrates sensitivity.
Listens to the patient.

Communication

| A | B | C | D | E |

Listening skills

| A | B | C | D | E |

Question framing

| A | B | C | D | E |

Verbal facilitation

| A | B | C | D | E |

⌘ Elicits relevant history, which may cover:

- types of substances used
- which substances are used regularly
- what pleasurable effects are obtained
- the amount of each drug consumed (in appropriate measures such as ounces)
- the duration of use, and duration of any period of abstinence
- symptoms on withdrawals from the drug and how he/she copes with them
- source of funding, such as shop-lifting, burglary
- route of use (oral, intramuscular, snorted or intravenous) and frequency
- are needles used? Where are they obtained from? Are needles shared? What sites are used for injection? Examine injection sites — is there evidence of recent use?
- when examining more private areas of the body, such as the inguinal area, it may be appropriate to ask for a chaperone to be present.
- if more than one drug is used at a time?
- is there a history of increasing tolerance to the effects of the drug, necessitating increases in amounts used?
- is there a history of deliberate or accidental overdoses? Was treatment needed for any episode?

⌘ Has the patient received any treatment, eg. substitute prescribing or toxification?

Diagnostic criteria | A | | B | | C | | D | | E | |

Factual knowledge | A | | B | | C | | D | | E | |

History | A | | B | | C | | D | | E | |

⌘ Elicits collateral history:

- contact with voluntary agencies, such as Narcotics or Alcoholics Anonymous
- has he/she been selling drugs?
- have there been any problems with the criminal justice system? Have there been any drug-related offences? Has the patient been subject to a Drug Treatment and Testing Order (DTTO)?
- history of imprisonment and probation? Any cautions or fines?
- are there any pending matters with the criminal justice system?

Collateral history | A | | B | | C | | D | | E | |

⌘ Assesses:

- impact of problems on family and friends.
- any physical complications, such as Hepatitis or HIV infection? Is the patient receiving any treatment, such as combination therapy for HIV
- has the patient developed comorbid mental illness, such as depression or psychosis?

Have you had any accidents or driving convictions related to your substance misuse?

⌘ Examines patient's motivation to change:

- why has the patient decided to give up drugs now?
- are any problems anticipated on giving up drug use?
- what preparation has the patient made towards this goal?
- what are the short- and long-term goals ?
- what kind of support networks does the patient have in the community?

Motivation | A | | B | | C | | D | | E | |

Patient's perception/the problem | A | | B | | C | | D | | E | |

Summarization | A | | B | | C | | D | | E | |

⌘ Explains the next stages of management, such as the need for further tests, eg. urine sample for toxicology screening and blood tests to check liver function. May have time to discuss substitute treatments, such as methadone or buprenorphine.

Global rating | A | | B | | C | | D | | E | |

6. Post-traumatic stress disorder

Establishes rapport, demonstrates sensitivity.
Appropriate empathy.
Asks open-ended and closed questions.
Listens to patient.
Allows the patient to talk freely.

Communication | A | | B | | C | | D | | E | |

Listening skills | A | | B | | C | | D | | E | |

⌘ Explores details of the accident, in particular the perceived severity.
⌘ Establishes the level of distress and fear at the time of the event.
⌘ Assesses symptom onset, duration and progress.
⌘ Assesses severity and frequency of current symptoms.
⌘ Assesses impact on activities of daily living and quality of life.

History | A | | B | | C | | D | | E | |

Verbal skills | A | | B | | C | | D | | E | |

Question framing | A | | B | | C | | D | | E | |

⌘ Explores flashbacks, occurring as recurrent images or thoughts. Establishes the intrusive nature of these thoughts/images, and frequency.
⌘ Explores nightmares and sleep difficulties.
⌘ Establishes nature and degree of avoidance symptoms.
⌘ Explores associated symptoms:

- mood disturbance, especially depression
- sleep and appetite problems
- loss of sense of enjoyment
- impaired concentration
- irritabilty
- emotional numbing
- thoughts or plans for suicide.

Emotional content   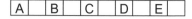 | A | | B | | C | | D | | E | |

Diagnostic criteria | A | | B | | C | | D | | E | |

Factual criteria | A | | B | | C | | D | | E | |

⌘ Other anxiety symptoms.
⌘ Current coping mechanisms, including drugs and alcohol.
⌘ Establishes the patient's expectations from this interview.

Summarization | A | | B | | C | | D | | E | |

Ending | A | | B | | C | | D | | E | |

Global rating | A | | B | | C | | D | | E | |

7. Alcohol dependence

Introduces self.
Explains purpose of the interview.
Empathises with patient and demonstrates sensitivity.
Asks open-ended and closed questions.
Establishes rapport and puts the patient at ease.

Introduction | A | | B | | C | | D | | E | |

Communication | A | | B | | C | | D | | E | |

Listening skills | A | | B | | C | | D | | E | |

Verbal skills | A | | B | | C | | D | | E | |

Use of language | A | | B | | C | | D | | E | |

⌘ Elicits relevant history, including:

- type of drink, frequency and amount consumed daily
- is he aware of how many units he drinks and what the recommended levels for 'safe' drinking are?
- has he made any attempt to control his drinking?
- have others made him aware of his problem with alcohol? How did he feel?
- has he ever felt guilty about his drinking?
- has he used alcohol as an 'eye-opener'?
- any recent period of abstinence?
- what happens when he is withdrawing from alcohol? How does he cope?
- does he feel a compulsion to drink, ie. does he crave alcohol?
- has he found himself drinking only certain types of drink for their alcohol content?

- has he found he needs increasing amounts to get the same effect?
- is most of his time spent in procuring, drinking and recovering from the effects of alcohol? Does alcohol take precedence over family and other pleasures?
- does he prefer to drink alone?
- has it affected his employment or relationships?
- does he drink despite knowing of the ill-effects of alcohol?
- has he had frequent relapses after periods of abstinence?

Dependence history   A   B   C   D   E

Factual content   A   B   C   D   E

Diagnostic criteria   A   B   C   D   E

⌘ Assesses the complications of alcohol dependence:

- any alcohol related memory problems?
- blackouts?
- falls?
- fits?
- haematemesis?
- melaena?
- loss of appetite?
- weight loss?

⌘ Explains what dependence means, and allows for questions.

Associated physical problems   A   B   C   D   E

Patient's concerns   A   B   C   D   E

Ending   A   B   C   D   E

Global rating   A   B   C   D   E

8. Depression/biological symptoms

⌘ Introduces self, explains reason for seeing a psychiatrist:

Hello Mr Rogers. My name is Dr Jones. I am one of the psychiatrists here. The doctor in casualty has asked me to speak to you, to see if there is anything we could help you with. He has been unable to find a cause for your chest pains but, on talking to you, thought your mood seemed a bit low.

Introduction   A   B   C   D   E

Listening skills	A	B	C	D	E

Verbal skills	A	B	C	D	E

Use of language	A	B	C	D	E

Clarifies the presenting complaints

⌘ Prevailing mood and changes recently:

> *How have you been feeling in yourself lately?*
> *Have you noticed a change in your mood recently?*

⌘ Explores associated changes in biological functions.
⌘ Energy levels and interest in normally pleasurable activities:

> *What about your energy levels?*
> *Have you been enjoying activities as much recently?*

⌘ Early morning waking/impaired appetite/weight loss:

> *How have you been sleeping?*
> *Do you have difficulty getting off to sleep?*

⌘ Impaired concentration:

> *How has your concentration been?*
> *Have you had any difficulty reading or watching television?*

⌘ Loss of libido:

> *What about your interest in sex? Has that been affected in any way?*
> *Have you lost interest in sex?*

History of mood change	A	B	C	D	E

Biological symptoms	A	B	C	D	E

⌘ Explores relevant medical history:

> *Have you had any serious physical illness, like diabetes, high blood pressure, or epilepsy? Have you had any operations or surgical procedures?*
> *Are you taking any prescribed medication currently? At what strength and how often?*
> *Approximately when did you start taking this medication?*
> *Have you had any problems with this medication?*

⌘ Explains that medication might contribute to or cause depressive symptoms:

The tablet you are taking for your high blood pressure can cause low mood in some people. Did your low mood start or become worse after you started the tablets?

Relevant medical history

A	B	C	D	E

Explores link between mood and medication

A	B	C	D	E

⌘ Summarises the findings and diagnosis, paying particular attention to the link between mental and physical problems.

The key point is to mention that he appears to have symptoms of **clinical** depression. Explain that this is more than just a simple low mood and is clearly affecting his capacity to enjoy his life, and also the routine functions of life like his sleep and appetite. In addition, you can state that depression can often present with physical symptoms like the chest pain he has been experiencing. Reassure him that you are not telling him that the pain is in his imagination, but that it could be related in some way to his depression (the 'mind-body link'). You could suggest that, although not all depression has an identifiable cause, in his case there may be link with his wife's being diagnosed with cancer. Mention that, although the symptoms of depression can be mimicked by certain medications, like his blood pressure tablets, it would not appear to be so in his case.

⌘ Conclude the interview in an appropriate manner, thanking the patient for his time and patience.

Summarization

A	B	C	D	E

Addresses patient's concerns

A	B	C	D	E

Ending

A	B	C	D	E

Global rating

A	B	C	D	E

9. Psychosexual history

⌘ Introduces self, explains reasons for appointment:

Hello Mr Smith. Thank you for attending this appointment. I am one of the psychiatrists here. Your GP asked for this appointment. I understand you had complained of difficulties in your relationship. I wonder if I could start off by talking to you about your recent relationships.

Introduction | A | B | C | D | E |

Listening skills | A | B | C | D | E |

Verbal facilitation | A | B | C | D | E |

⌘ Elicits a psychosexual history. This is an area which, though daunting, is commonly not enquired about in much depth. It is easier to start by acknowledging that this might be a very personal area to talk about:

> *Some of the next few questions are personal, and you might not wish to answer them. They might, however, help me to get a clearer picture of your lifestyle, and the various pressures you face everyday. I'd like to start by asking you about your sexual orientation, that is whether you are heterosexual or otherwise.*

- you could ask at what age he attained puberty, had his first relationship, and first sexual intercourse
- you will need to ask about number of sexual partners, relationships, their duration, and the main reason for breaking up. Also ask about unprotected sex, and intravenous drug use
- any paraphilias:

> *Do you have any unusual sexual interests or fetishes?*

⌘ Previous tests for sexually transmitted infections:

> *Have you had blood tests for sexually transmitted infections, like HIV, hepatitis, herpes, syphilis, or gonorrhoea? Have you suffered from any infections in the genital area like thrush or warts? Have you received any treatment for any of these? What about your partner?*

History | A | B | C | D | E |

Verbal skills | A | B | C | D | E |

Question framing | A | B | C | D | E |

⌘ You will need to discuss the current state of his relationship(s), and whether his partner is supportive or not?

> *Are you currently in a relationship? Are you married, separated or divorced?*
> *Is your partner helpful and supportive towards you? Do you get on with him/her?*

⌘ Lifestyle and relationship factors:

> *How long have you been in this relationship? Have you had previous relationships? What was the longest? Have you had any short-term relationships or 'one-night stands?' Have you had unprotected sex with any of these partners? What about your current partner? Do you have any children — ages, where they are, and who they live with.*

Verbal skills | A | B | C | D | E |

Question framing | A | B | C | D | E |

Sensitivity and non-judgemental manner | A | B | C | D | E |

⌘ Summarize the main points in the history and ends the interview appropriately.

⌘ The key point here is to reflect back his reasons for taking the overdose and how it appears that this was an impulsive act in the context of alcohol abuse.

⌘ The other point is to mention any specific risk factors you may have picked up in the psychosexual history. It is likely that he will still be concerned about having an infection. Address this directly:

> *I can understand that you might still be concerned about whether you have caught anything nasty or not. I can give you the number of the local GUM clinic where they can first discuss your concerns in greater depth, perhaps give you a clearer picture of the actual rather than imagined risks and also test you for sexually transmitted infections. For some tests like the HIV test, they will usually offer you specific pre-test and post-test counselling.*

⌘ End the interview by thanking him for his time and patience.

Summarization | A | B | C | D | E |

Addresses patient's concerns | A | B | C | D | E |

Ending | A | B | C | D | E |

Global rating | A | B | C | D | E |

10. Anxiety

Introduces self.
Explains reason for the interview.
Establishes rapport.
Is sensitive to patient's difficulties.

Uses a mixture of open and closed questions.

Listening skills

| A | | B | | C | | D | | E | |

Use of language

| A | | B | | C | | D | | E | |

Emotional content

| A | | B | | C | | D | | E | |

⌘ Explores:

- mood
- anxiety
- precipitating factors
- beliefs
- behaviours
- other physical symptoms.

Exploration of presenting complaint

⌘ Gives appropriate information about her presentation:

- she is probably experiencing panic attacks
- a panic attack often presents with the physical symptoms she has described
- influence of stressors, like her father's death and arguments with husband
- role of hyperventilation in production of symptoms
- maintaining role of anxiety and fear of serious illness
- risk of using avoidance as a coping mechanism.

Giving information

| A | | B | | C | | D | | E | |

⌘ Gives suggestions to address the problem:

- develop insight in the mechanisms that play a role
- re-breathing
- controlled breathing
- relaxation
- cognitive behavioural therapy
- antidepressants, in particular the SSRIs
- benzodiazepines, with a caution about disadvantages.

Discusses treatment

| A | | B | | C | | D | | E | |

Summarization

| A | | B | | C | | D | | E | |

Global rating

| A | | B | | C | | D | | E | |

11. Lack of energy and paranoia

Establishes rapport.
Balances open and closed questions.
Avoids jargon.

Listening skills |A| |B| |C| |D| |E| |

Question framing |A| |B| |C| |D| |E| |

Use of language |A| |B| |C| |D| |E| |

⌘ Uses appropriate questions in order to explore presenting complaint:

- what the main problems are
- duration of presenting complaints
- progression of symptoms
- precipitating factors
- alcohol and drug use
- other psychotic symptoms
- mood.

Exploration of presenting complaint |A| |B| |C| |D| |E| |

⌘ Points out that cannabis use can lead to apathy, lack of motivation and memory problems.

⌘ Explains that excessive cannabis use can also cause psychotic symptoms.

⌘ Addresses risks when driving and physical risks from smoking such as cancer.

⌘ Is non-judgemental and presents information objectively.

⌘ Information about risks and side-effects.

⌘ Explains that cannabis is not legal, though it has been reclassified from a class B to a class C drug. The police have adopted a policy not to arrest people for individual use, but could still do so if there are other reasons.

Legal issues |A| |B| |C| |D| |E| |

Global rating |A| |B| |C| |D| |E| |

12. Sleeping difficulties

Explains the purpose of the meeting.
Establishes rapport.
Follows a logical line of questioning.
Asks open and closed questions.

Listening skills

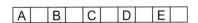

Question framing

⌘ Takes a sleep history:

> *At what time do you usually go to bed?*
> *How long does it take you to fall asleep?*
> *Do you read, listen to music or watch TV while in bed?*
> *What do you do when you can't sleep?*
> *Do you have a bedtime routine? Can you describe what you do?*
> *When do have your last meal of the day?*
> *Do you drink coffee, tea, cola or alcohol in the evening?*
> *What about the environment around where you live. Is it noisy?*
> *Does anything keep you awake at night like an uncomfortable bed, pain or noise?*

Sleep history

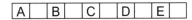

⌘ Explains about the factors that may influence her ability to sleep, such as having a late meal, drinking cola, watching TV in bed, a noisy room and excessive worrying.

⌘ Gives suggestions for interventions.

Explanations and interventions

⌘ Explains risks of benzodiazepines:

- risk of dependence
- not for long term use
- risk of sedation the next day
- influence on driving skills.

Risks of benzodiazepines

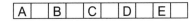

⌘ Gives suggestions for alternative approaches, for instance:

- sleep hygiene
- relaxation

- use of tapes
- measures like warm milk
- other medication.

Treatment
A	B	C	D	E

Global rating
A	B	C	D	E

13. Grief

Introduces self.
Shows empathy and understanding.
Is patient and sensitive to patient's feelings.

Introduction
A	B	C	D	E

Listening skills
A	B	C	D	E

Verbal skills
A	B	C	D	E

Use of language
A	B	C	D	E

⌘ Explores circumstances of wife's death:

- how she passed away
- how long ago
- how old was she when she died
- whether her death was expected or sudden
- where was the patient at the time:

    Were you able to say goodbye?
    Did you see the body?

History
A	B	C	D	E

⌘ Explores possibility of typical (in terms of intensity or duration) grief:

How do you feel about the loss? Do you sometimes feel as if it has not actually happened? Have you been able to express your pain/grief? **or** *Have you cried? Can you talk about it? Do you feel things are changing:*
    ~ are you making any progress?
    ~ do you feel you are stuck?
    ~ do you have an interest in anything?
    ~ are you able to move on?
    ~ do you feel your life is still worth living?

Signs of typical grief | A | | B | | C | | D | | E | |

Asks about factors related to atypical grief

⌘ Duration of marriage, and what kind of a person his wife was:

> *Can you tell me about your wife?*
> *What kind of person was she? Did you get on?*
> *What was your relationship like?*
> *How did you deal with your wife's hectic social life?*

⌘ Any other bereavements lately.

⌘ Any early losses in your life.

Signs of atypical grief | A | | B | | C | | D | | E | |

Risk factors | A | | B | | C | | D | | E | |

⌘ Gives suggestions for further action and further support:

- explanation that a lot of his experiences are understandable and not unusual
- role that his daughters are playing in taking care of him
- other contacts, that could play a supportive role, like neighbours, friends, the Church, and support from his GP
- bereavement counselling from external agencies, such as CRUSE.
- role of medication, with limitations.

Management | A | | B | | C | | D | | E | |

Global score | A | | B | | C | | D | | E | |

Section two:
Examination skills

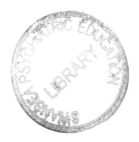

Instructions for candidates

14. Frontal lobe function

This fifty-six-year-old man presented to his GP with lack of initiative and inappropriate, disinhibited behaviour, which is quite out of character for him.

Test his frontal lobe functions.

15. Capacity to refuse consent to treatment

This twenty-six-year-old heroin addict has been injecting himself in the groin. He has developed localised cellulitis and attended the A&E Department. The surgical SHO who saw him advised to come into hospital for a course of intravenous antibiotics. Initially, he agreed to this plan, but he has now changed his mind and wants to take his own discharge.

You are asked to assess whether he has the capacity to refuse treatment.

16. Risk assessment of a suicidal patient

You are called to see this thirty-six-year-old lady by the casualty medical officer (CMO) at your local district general hospital. The CMO is concerned about this patient and thinks she is depressed and suicidal. The patient has complained of feeling hopeless.

Assess the suicidal risk posed by this patient.

17. Assessment for akathisia

You are called to see this nineteen-year-old young man admitted for the first time onto a psychiatric ward. The working diagnosis is of an acute psychotic disorder. He was commenced on oral haloperidol a day after his admission. He now complains of restlessness and feeling agitated.

Take a history, and assess for akathisia.

18. Insight/attitude

You are asked to review a patient on the acute admissions ward. She is a nineteen-year-old girl, who was attending college until eighteen months ago. She had been brought into the A&E department last night after jumping out of the first floor window of her parents' house. She was admitted as a voluntary patient on the ward after she admitted experiencing command hallucinations telling her to kill herself. She refused all medication last night. This morning she has tried to leave the ward.

Assess this patient's insight into her illness and her attitude to treatment. If you decide to detain her under Section 5(2) of the Mental Health Act 1983, how would you proceed?

19. Eating disorder

You are asked to see a twenty-three-year-old lady in the out-patient clinic. She works as a manager in a gym, and has been referred by her GP who is concerned at her weight loss. She has lost five stone in weight in less than a year, and in the last four weeks has been eating only two apples a day. At her last consultation with him, she asked for a prescription of laxatives.

Assess this patient for symptoms and signs of anorexia.

20. Thyroid

You are asked to see a thirty-five-year-old lady in the out-patient clinic, who has been treated by her GP for depression over the last three years. Although her mood has lifted a little, she still complains that it is low at times. The GP note mentions that she has put on some weight in the last year, and that she complains of being tired at every appointment. He has also started treating her recently for diagnosed hypertension.

Take a brief medical history and examine the patient for signs of thyroid disease.

21. First rank symptoms

Assess this thirty-year-old man for first rank symptoms of schizophrenia.

22. Suicidal intent

A fifty-two-year-old man has taken an overdose of paracetamol. He was taken to A&E by a neighbour. You have been asked to see him.

Assess his suicidal intent.

23. Personality

This twenty-four-year-old woman has taken an overdose of fluoxetine. The liaison nurse has already completed an assessment with regards to the overdose.

You have been asked to obtain some information about her personality.

24. Mini Mental State Examination

This seventy-one-year-old man has been referred to you. His family have noticed that he has become slightly forgetful over the last six months.

Assess his cognitive functioning using the MMSE.

2.2

Instructions for actors

14. Frontal lobe function

You are a fifty-six-year-old man who has developed a change in behaviour due to an abnormality in the brain. You have become apathetic and do not care about your appearance and your manners. When asked to say as many objects in one minute as you can, you only come up with six, and you then repeat some a few times. You cannot explain the meaning of proverbs and give unlikely answers when asked to give estimates of size or number.

15. Capacity to refuse consent to treatment

You are a heroin addict, and have been injecting it for the last ten years. You are not physically well. Once the veins in your arms were damaged from frequent injections, you started injecting into a vein in your groin. You now have an infection at the injection site in your groin. At the local A&E department, the doctor explains that you need antibiotics in an intravenous drip. You agree to be admitted onto a medical ward to have the antibiotics. Later, you change your mind because you want to leave to get another 'fix' of heroin.

You understand that you need antibiotics to treat your infection and that it needs to be given slowly via the drip. You know that the infection may get worse and that you could become seriously ill. You ask for the antibiotic in tablet form, even though you are aware that they may not be as effective. You are increasingly impatient and keep asking when you can go.

16. Risk assessment of a suicidal patient

You are a thirty-six-year-old mother of two young children. Six months ago you separated from your long-term partner. Since then, you have had recurrent headaches, body aches, low energy levels, and poor concentration. You've been feeling depressed, with impaired sleep and poor appetite, and have been neglecting your children. You have had thoughts of jumping in front of a moving car. Yesterday, you stood by the road side for two hours, before your children persuaded you to return home. You have taken two impulsive overdoses of paracetamol in the last two months, both at times when you were drunk. You did not tell any one about them and slept them off. Tonight, you do not think you will be safe at home. You have no friends locally and no other support in looking after your children. You are desperate for help.

17. Assessment for akathisia

You are a nineteen-year-old student on a computer course. Lately, you have been feeling as if the Ministry of Defence has been trying to have you murdered. You get messages warning you about this from the newspaper and television. You had to drop out of college. When you were admitted to a psychiatric unit for the first time last week, you agreed to take some medication to help you feel calmer.

However, since you started on the tablets, you have been feeling even more restless, and your muscles have been tense. This has become so bad that you now think that you might try to kill yourself just to try and escape these unpleasant feelings. You are quite certain that the medication has brought this on, and that it has become a lot worse since this morning. You are unable to sit still and have to keep pacing around the room as the interview progresses.

18. Insight/attitude

You are a nineteen-year-old girl who has been hearing voices for the last three years, mostly calling you names and telling you that 'they' are going to kill you. You have been trying to cope but had to drop out of college when the voices became too intrusive. Last night, they started shouting at you again, telling you to kill yourself. You tried to escape from them by jumping out of your bedroom window. You were admitted voluntarily on a psychiatric ward for observation. Although you were offered medication to calm you down and help with the voices, you have refused it as you think it might have been poisoned. You tried to leave hospital as you heard the same voices threatening you on the ward. The nurses now want you to speak with the psychiatrist, because you are insisting on leaving.

19. Eating disorder

You are a twenty-three-year-old female manager of a gym. Your GP has asked you to see a psychiatrist after you asked for laxatives to help you lose weight. You have already lost five stone in weight in the last year, and have cut down your food intake to just two apples a day in the last month. You have been trying to lose weight by over-exercising in the gym, and have recently started making yourself sick after every meal. You still consider yourself 'fat' and would like to lose some more weight. You have had dizzy spells in the last week, and your periods stopped about a year ago.

20. Thyroid

You are a thirty-five-year-old lady, who has been referred by your GP because he wants a second opinion in treating your depression. For the last three years you have been feeling low in yourself, with episodes of crying, and a persisting tiredness. The antidepressants you have been on have helped a little. You are now sleeping a bit better. However, over the last year, you have put on two stone in weight despite no major change in your diet. Your GP has also told you that you have high blood pressure and has started you on treatment for this.

21. First rank symptoms

You are a thirty-year-old man, who lives alone in a flat. You think that you can hear the neighbours talking about you in the next door flat. They say things like, 'he is a bastard', and, 'he is a paedophile'. They have been commenting on your actions since you first heard them. More recently, they have been making threats to kill you.

You also feel that strangers on the street are able somehow to know what you are thinking. You think they may be using some kind of microwave device, because you have heard about this sort of thing on the television. You have no other unusual thoughts.

22. Suicidal intent after an overdose

You are a fifty-two-year-old bank manager, who was divorced from your wife of thirty years last December. You have two daughters, one of whom lives locally. You live alone in a three-bedroomed house. Recently, you were told that you have lung cancer and have been told that you do not have long to live as the cancer has spread throughout your body.

Two days ago, you took an overdose of around sixty paracetamol tablets at home. You did not expect to be found, but were discovered by a worried neighbour. You have been thinking about taking an overdose for about a week. You did not mention it to anybody. You intended to die, so that you would not have to go through the suffering of a long and possibly painful terminal illness. You expected that the overdose would kill you, despite medical attention. You had written a suicide note to your daughters and ex-wife. Now, you regret that your plan did not work, because the situation you find yourself in has not changed at all.

23. Personality

You are a twenty-four-year-old woman, who has taken an overdose of twenty tablets of an antidepressant. You have been living with your boyfriend for the last three months, but the relationship has been volatile. Three days ago you found out that he has been seeing another woman. You took the overdose this morning and told him about it immediately. You have been out of work for the last few months, after quitting jobs in a pub and a factory. You have had several short-term relationships, none lasting for longer than three months.

You have been feeling depressed on and off ever since your teens. You have felt suicidal at times, and say you wanted to kill yourself when you took this overdose. You do not feel suicidal at present. You have taken two overdoses in the past, both times when you were going through a difficult patch in a relationship. You have never harmed yourself in any other way. You smoke cannabis regularly and drink large amounts of alcohol, mainly at the weekends. You have been in trouble with the police twice for being drunk and disorderly. You have never felt paranoid and do not hear voices.

You had a difficult childhood. Your parents divorced when you were five years old. Your mother remarried, but you did not get on with your stepfather. You did reasonably well at school, but did not have many friends and as a result were bullied throughout. You are not very confident and find it very difficult to be on your own.

24. Mini Mental State Examination

You are a seventy-one-year-old man, with an increasingly poor memory. Your family have brought you to see a psychiatrist. When taking the test you give wrong answers when asked about the date and the day of the week. When asked to recall three words you have learned earlier, you can only remember two. Otherwise you are advised to act as normal.

Please follow instructions given to you by the candidate.

2.3

Instructions for examiners

---

1. Frontal lobe function

Introduces self.
Is patient and sensitive to the patient's difficulties.
Introduces the tests and explains the procedure clearly.

Consent | A | | B | | C | | D | | E |

Explanation | A | | B | | C | | D | | E |

Use of language | A | | B | | C | | D | | E |

⌘ Tests verbal fluency:

- F, A and S test (name as many words starting with the letters 'F', 'A' and 'S' as you can)
- animal, fruit or supermarket fluency test.

Each test for one minute.

Tests verbal fluency | A | | B | | C | | D | | E |

⌘ Tests abstraction by asking patient to explain proverbs like:

- don't judge a book by its cover', 'still waters run deep', 'a bird in hand is worth two in the bush', or 'one swallow does not a summer make.'

⌘ Asks patient to explain differences and similarities between words, such as:

- apple and banana
- table and chair
- glass and ice
- mistake and lie
- poem and statue
- praise and punishment.

⌘ Asks patient to make estimates, such as:

How fast does a horse gallop?

What is the height of an average English woman?
How many camels are there in Holland?

Tests of abstract thinking | A | | B | | C | | D | | E | |

⌘ Tests for response inhibition and set shifting:

- asks patient to finish a sequence of alternating squares and triangles
- asks patient to perform the Luria three-step test (placing a fist, then edge of the palm, and then a flat palm onto the palm of the opposite hand, and repeating the sequence)
- asks patient to perform the Luria three-step test
- trail making test (connect numbers and letters, such as '1' to 'A', then to '2', then to 'B', then to '3', and finally to 'C').

⌘ Tests frontal lobe release signs (primitive reflexes), for example:

- grasping reflex — strokes patient's palm while distracting the patient, and watches for involuntary grasping which can be subtle
- pouting reflex — taps on a spatula placed on patient's lips, resulting in pouting
- glabellar tap — taps between the eyebrows, which causes repeated blinking even after five or more taps.

Response-inhibition and set shifting | A | | B | | C | | D | | E | |

Tests for reflexes | A | | B | | C | | D | | E | |

Summarization | A | | B | | C | | D | | E | |

Global rating | A | | B | | C | | D | | E | |

15. Capacity to refuse consent to treatment

Establishes rapport.
Is respectful and sensitive to the patient's situation.
Explains the reason for the assessment.
Starts with asking open questions.

Consent | A | | B | | C | | D | | E | |

Explanation | A | | B | | C | | D | | E | |

Listening skills | A | | B | | C | | D | | E | |

Question framing | A | | B | | C | | D | | E | |

⌘ Obtain background information:

- whether in a relationship or not at the moment
- domestic situation
- duration of dependence on heroin
- use of other drugs or alcohol.

⌘ Establishes reasons for refusal to accept treatment and wish to leave.

Obtaining background information |A| |B| |C| |D| |E| |

⌘ Establishes whether he understands and retains information about:

- the medical problem (what problem do you have right now?)
- the proposed treatment — what is involved in the treatment
- alternatives to the proposed treatment
- the consequences when treatment is refused:

  What could happen if you don't have the antibiotic? Would you become more ill? Would you be placing your life at risk without it?

Assesses understanding and retention |A| |B| |C| |D| |E| |
of information

⌘ Establishes whether he believes the information given about the need for treatment and also whether he is able to weigh his options in balance to come to a decision:

  Why have you decided to refuse treatment?
  Why have you changed your mind about staying in hospital? Is anything worrying you in hospital?

⌘ Assesses mood.

Assesses ability to weigh up information |A| |B| |C| |D| |E| |
and come to a decision

⌘ Concludes by asking whether the patient would like to discuss his decision further or has any questions.

Formulating conclusion |A| |B| |C| |D| |E| |

Global rating |A| |B| |C| |D| |E| |

16. Risk assessment of a suicidal patient

Ensures patient is in a quiet room.
Introduces himself/herself.
Explains the purpose of assessment.
Listens to patient, allows the patient to talk.
Empathises.

Introduction

| A | B | C | D | E | |

Communication

| A | B | C | D | E | |

Listening skills

| A | B | C | D | E | |

⌘ Explores hopelessness, low mood.

⌘ Allows patient to interrupt.

⌘ Detailed history of suicidal ideation and planning:

> *Do you get any pleasure out of life? Do you find it hard to see a day through?*
> *Is life stressful or a burden? How hopeful are you from day-to-day?*
> *Do you wish it would all end?* **or** *Have you had thoughts of ending it all?*
> **or** *Have you ever thought of ending your life?*
> *Have you thought how you might do it? Have you made any plans? How far have you gone with your plans?*
> *Have you told anyone about these thoughts?*
> *Have you written a suicide note? Have you written a will?*
> *Could anything stop you from proceeding with your plans?*
> *Is there anything to live for?*

These suggested questions can be complimented with screening questions on depression, which are covered in *1.3, pages 20–22.*

⌘ Checks medical history of headaches.

⌘ Gives explanation about depression.

⌘ Highlights the need for inpatient assessment.

History and severity

| A | B | C | D | E | |

Verbal facilitation

| A | B | C | D | E | |

Question framing

| A | B | C | D | E | |

Use of language | A | B | C | D | E |

Emotional content | A | B | C | D | E |

⌘ Explores:

- signs of depression
- seriousness of intent
- degree of preoccupation of suicidality
- hopelessness
- any previous attempts?
- deterrents/protective factors
- reasons why patient feels unsafe to go home
- reasons for seeking help on this occassion
- the headaches
- patient's expectations from the interview
- care arrangements for children (consider child protection issues).

Have you tried to harm yourself previously? In what way? On how many occaions? Could you tell me more about the last time you harmed yourself? Have you been able to distract yourself from these thoughts? If so, how? What sorts of things help when you have these thoughts? Do you feel that you have enough control over your actions? How likely do you think you are to kill yourself? Are you hopeful for the future? How can we help you? What are your expectations of this assessment?

Explores risk factors | A | B | C | D | E |

Explores protective factors | A | B | C | D | E |

Factual content | A | B | C | D | E |

Addresses patient's concerns | A | B | C | D | E |

Ending | A | B | C | D | E |

Global rating | A | B | C | D | E |

Assessment for akathisia

Initial discussion with examiner about steps taken prior to interview:

1. Read through medical notes and speak with nursing staff to get a clear picture of initial presentation and observations since admission
2. Previous history of restlessness and complaints of muscular tension.

3. Evidence of previous suicidal ideation or attempts.
4. History of illicit drug use.
5. Treatment for current medical conditions.
6. Treatment with specific drugs such as anti-emetics.
7. Ideally, ask for an escort and conduct interview in a quiet room.

⌘ Introduces self and explains reasons for interview:

> *Good morning, I am Dr Jones, one of the psychiatrists looking after you.*
> *The nurses on the ward have asked me to see you. I understand you have*
> *had some worries about your medication. What seems to be the problem?*

Communication with examiner | A | B | C | D | E |

Communication with patient | A | B | C | D | E |

⌘ Facilitates interview:

- allows patient to verbalise his concerns fully
- avoids interruption
- focuses on patient's main concerns
- clarifies the onset, duration, and progression of symptoms, as well as aggravating and relieving factors
- enquires about related mood and explores suicidal ideations in detail
- examines relationship between starting the new medication and onset of symptoms
- notes the nature of any abnormal movements and objectively assesses the degree of restlessness.

Candidate observation and examination | A | B | C | D | E |

⌘ Detailed screen for akathisia symptoms:

> *How long have you been suffering from this problem?*
> *What's the longest you can sit down for? How difficult is it to settle down in*
> *one place?*
> *Do you feel tense? Are you able to relax at all?*
> *What have you tried to help relieve your distress?*
> *Which parts of your body are affected?*
> *Is this an ongoing problem or is it intermittent? Do you feel like this only*
> *when you are at rest? Or does it also occur when you are moving around?*
> *Does your movement make it worse or relieve it? Is it affected by the*
> *position of your body or limbs?*
> *Is it affected by environment, temperature or your emotional state?*
> *Is it altered in any way when you close your eyes?*
> *Have the staff noticed it when you are asleep?*
> *Are you aware of your own restlessness? Can you describe it for me?*

Several of the features described can also be discreetly observed during the course of the interview.

⌘ Advises the patient:

> *From what I have read and heard from staff, and my own observations of you during our chat, I think you are experiencing a side-effect of the medication you are on. This side-effect is called 'akathisia' and usually occurs early in the course of treatment. We can try to make it better by decreasing the dose of the medication or we can change you over to another drug less likely to cause this side-effect. Let me have a word with my supervising consultant and get back to you about what we can do to help. In the meantime, I can prescribe a drug called procyclidine to help with the problem. I need to ask you a few more questions about your medical history just to make sure I can give it to you safely.*

Candidate feedback to patient |A| |B| |C| |D| |E| |

⌘ Advice to accompanying staff (which you could address to the examiner).

⌘ Advice on placing the patient under constant observation in view of the distress he has expressed and his admission of suicidal thoughts.

Advice to staff |A| |B| |C| |D| |E| |

Global rating |A| |B| |C| |D| |E| |

> It is useful to keep in mind a general definition of akathisia as, a subjective feeling of muscular tension, secondary to treatment with antipsychotics, that presents as restlessness, pacing about, and being unable to sit still, and which can be easily mistaken for psychotic agitation.

18. Insight/attitude

Introduces self and explains purpose of interview.
It is important at the start to engage with the patient and to establish some rapport, as it seems that she is already paranoid and may be reluctant to talk:

> *I understand you have tried to leave hospital. The nursing staff have asked me to talk to you because they are concerned for you. Could you perhaps tell me why you want to leave?*

The patient may choose to talk about her reasons for wanting to leave or not. The key point is to establish some rapport that will permit you to ask further, more detailed questions.

Introduction	A	B	C	D	E

Listening skills	A	B	C	D	E

Use of language	A	B	C	D	E

Establishes rapport	A	B	C	D	E

Elicits the main components of insight including:

⌘ Acknowledging that something is actually being experienced/perceived:

> *Has anything unusual, that you can't explain, happened to you lately?* **or** *Have you been hearing or seeing anything unusual that you can't explain?*

⌘ Admitting that these experiences are not 'normal':

> *Do you think that the average person on the street hears voices the way you have described to me?* **or** *Would you expect that the average person on the street experiences the same things that you have been experiencing lately?*

⌘ Acknowledges that these experiences might be part of a mental illness:

> *Is it possible that what you are experiencing is, in fact, part of a mental illness?* **or** *Could it be that your experiences are part of an illness affecting your mind?*

⌘ Believing that assistance of some kind is needed to help with the problem:

> *Do you feel you need help to deal with this problem?*
> *What kind of help do you think would be useful?*

Verbal facilitation	A	B	C	D	E

Explores the components of insight	A	B	C	D	E

Non-judgemental and demonstrates sensitivity	A	B	C	D	E

⌘ Assesses attitude to treatment:

> *I understand that you refused the medication you were offered last night. Could you tell me if there was any particular reason why? Is there any other way in which you think we can help you?*

This will help to decide whether or not the patient consents to staying in hospital and taking medication. If she is making an attempt to leave and you consider there is a risk to her own health or safety or for the protection of others, you may need to detain her under the powers of Section 5(2) of the Mental Health Act. Attitude to treatment at this stage can influence prognosis in the long term, because it will effect the extent of her engagement with services and treatment.

⌘ Looks at the broader picture of attitude to the psychiatric services:

> *How do you feel about being here on this ward? Do you think it has helped you to be here? Would you agree to stay on the ward to allow us time to get to know you better and find out how we can best help you?*

⌘ Contrasts the pros and cons of her particular attitude to treatment:

> *Let's look at the good (helpful) and bad (unhelpful) points about the options that you have in front of you. Perhaps we could make this into a table, to make it easier to understand and remember.*

Explores non-compliance | A | | B | | C | | D | | E | |

Assesses attitude to treatment | A | | B | | C | | D | | E | |

⌘ Summarizes his/her opinion about the patient's presentation and discusses the reasons for detention.

⌘ Ending this interview is particularly difficult. From the way the question is worded it would appear that she refuses to stay on the ward. You will need to explain about your detaining her in hospital:

> *Thank you for taking the time to answer my questions. As you know, I have looked carefully at your medical notes and have also talked with the nursing staff. We are concerned about what happened to you last night, your trying to leave and also about what you are saying now. I think it would be safer for you to stay in hospital, where we can get to know you better, and help you by treating what we think is a mental illness. In view of our concerns for your safety, your previous attempt to leave and your insistence on leaving now, I am afraid I have to make a recommendation for you to be detained here against your will under Section 5(2) of the Mental Health Act 1983. This is a piece of law that applies to patients in hospital and it allows for you to be detained here for up to seventy-two hours for further observation. Well before that period of time has elapsed, two doctors (one of whom is independent) and an approved social worker will see you again to decide on whether you need to stay in hospital any longer. I am going to give you a leaflet which explains in more detail what I have done and what your rights are. If you have any questions, please let me or one of the nurses know.*

Summarization | A | B | C | D | E |

Communicating bad news | A | B | C | D | E |

Ending | A | B | C | D | E |

Global rating | A | B | C | D | E |

19. Eating disorder

Introduces self, and explains reason for meeting with a psychiatrist:

> *Hello, Mrs Brown. Your GP has asked me to meet with you to look at some aspects of your physical health, and in particular his concerns about your weight. Could we perhaps start by talking about how you have been feeling in yourself lately?*

The key point to remember is that she may not understand why she needs to talk to a psychiatrist and she may not be too forthcoming if you launch into questions about her eating problems right at the beginning. Once you have established some rapport, you can ask more focused questions

Introduction | A | B | C | D | E |

Establishes rapport | A | B | C | D | E |

Tactful questioning | A | B | C | D | E |

⌘ Ascertains whether the classical triad of weight loss, morbid fear of fatness, and secondary amenorrhoea are present:

> *How have you been eating lately? Have you been putting on or losing weight lately? Do you know what you weigh at the moment? What is your height?*
> *What is your ideal weight? How hard have you been trying to achieve it? Have you been scared of putting on any weight? Would you consider yourself 'fat'?*
> *Have your periods been affected at all?*

⌘ Ascertains daily dietary intake:

> *Could you run through an average day with me, listing what you eat during the course of each meal?*

Diagnostic criteria　　　　　　|A| |B| |C| |D| |E| |

Factual knowledge　　　　　　|A| |B| |C| |D| |E| |

⌘ Elicits what measures have been taken to lose weight:

> *What sorts of things have you been doing to keep your weight down?*
> *Have you been exercising more than usual or using laxatives or water pills?*
> *Have you been making yourself sick? How often?*

⌘ Elicits associated mood and biological symptoms:

> *How has your mood been with all these changes in your weight? When your*
> *mood has been particularly low, have you had thoughts of wanting to end it*
> *all? Have you acted on any of these thoughts?*
> *How have you been sleeping? Has your concentration been affected? For*
> *example, have you been able to watch television or read the newspaper?*

⌘ Elicits history of impulsivity in other areas.

⌘ Elicits weight control measures.

⌘ Explores comorbid symptoms.

⌘ Physical examination:

- calculate current BMI (weight in kg/height in m^2)
- head to toe examination focusing on the presence or not of Lanugo hair, pallor/carotenemia, bilateral parotid enlargement, erosion of the teeth, signs of vitamin deficiencies such as bald tongue, loss of secondary sexual characteristics, Russell's sign (erosion of dorsal surface of knuckles), arrhythmias, muscle wasting.

Obtains consent　　　　　　　|A| |B| |C| |D| |E| |

Explains procedure　　　　　　|A| |B| |C| |D| |E| |

Performs relevant physical examination |A| |B| |C| |D| |E| |

Ending　　　　　　　　　　　　|A| |B| |C| |D| |E| |

Global rating　　　　　　　　　|A| |B| |C| |D| |E| |

20. Thyroid

Introduces self and explains the reasons for examination.

Introduction |A| |B| |C| |D| |E| |

Establishes rapport |A| |B| |C| |D| |E| |

⌘ Elicits medical history, starting with significant medical illnesses:

> *Have you had any medical illnesses, like diabetes, high blood pressure, or epilepsy? Have you had any injuries, or accidents? Have you ever injured your head, or lost consciousness? Have you ever had to be admitted to hospital? What was it for?*
> *Could I ask about your periods? When did you last have one? Do you think there's any chance you could be pregnant?*
> *Have you ever had any major operations?*
> *Are you on any medication for your physical problems? What is it called? How often do you take your medication?*
> *Are you taking any other, non-prescribed medication?*

Listening skills |A| |B| |C| |D| |E| |

Use of language |A| |B| |C| |D| |E| |

Elicits relevant medical history |A| |B| |C| |D| |E| |

⌘ Systematically elaborates on the major complaints:

> *Have you had any complaints of a physical nature?*
> *Tell me about your cough? When did it start? Did it come on gradually or did it start suddenly? How has it progressed over time? Tell me how it is now?*

⌘ As there is a clue that this is a thyroid case, focus on some important physical symptoms:

> *Have you put on any weight recently? Has your appetite been any different? Have you been feeling tired at all? Have you found yourself disliking the cold weather more than usual? Have you noticed any change in the quality of your voice?* **or** *Is your voice more hoarse than usual?*
> *Have you noticed any swelling around your neck? Have you noticed any swelling up of your hands, feet, or eyelids? Have you noticed any pain in your wrists, or tingling down one side of either hand?*

Explores primary symptoms | A | B | C | D | E |

Explores comorbid symptoms | A | B | C | D | E |

⌘ Performs relevant physical examination:

- Look for pallor, dry flaky skin and hair, alopecia, purplish lips, malar flush, carotinaemia, myxoedema (non-pittting oedema, usually seen in the skin of the hands, feet, and eyelids, where it presents as periorbital puffiness), low-pitched voice, slurred speech due to enlarged tongue, bradycardia, hypertension, congestive cardiac failure, delayed relaxation of deep tendon reflexes, and carpal tunnel syndrome.

Obtains consent | A | B | C | D | E |

Explains procedure | A | B | C | D | E |

Performs relevant physical examination | A | B | C | D | E |

Ending | A | B | C | D | E |

Global rating | A | B | C | D | E |

21. First rank symptoms

Introduces self and explains the need to ask questions.
Establishes rapport.
Is sensitive to patient's feelings.

Introduction | A | B | C | D | E |

Listening skills | A | B | C | D | E |

Verbal skills | A | B | C | D | E |

Use of language | A | B | C | D | E |

⌘ Asks introductory questions like:

Do you feel anything strange is going on? **or** *Do you ever feel as if something is going on around you without your knowledge?*
Has anything happened to you lately that you can't explain?

Asks for further details and clarification

⌘ Third person hallucinations:

> *Do you ever hear peoples' voices when there is nobody around?*
> *Do you ever hear voices when you are on your own?*
> *What do they say?*
> *Can you give me an example?*

⌘ Hallucinations in the form of a commentary:

> *Do you ever hear voices commenting on what you are doing?*
> *Do you ever hear voices talk about what you are doing at the time?*
> *Do you hear a running commentary of your actions?*

⌘ Hearing thoughts spoken out loud:

> *Do you hear your thoughts being spoken out aloud?*
> *Can other people hear your thoughts?*

Elicits auditory hallucinations | A | | B | | C | | D | | E | |

⌘ Thought withdrawal or insertion:

> *Is any external agency interfering with your thoughts?*
> *Are your thoughts not wholly your own?*
> *Is anybody putting thoughts into your head?*
> *Is anyone taking thoughts out of your head? Can you tell me how?*

⌘ Thought broadcasting:

> *Are your thoughts broadcast to others?*
> *Do others know your thoughts?*
> *Is there anything like telepathy going on?*

Thought interference | A | | B | | C | | D | | E | |

⌘ Delusional perception:

> *Have you experienced anything that made you understand that something was going on around you?* **or** *Has anything happened that made you suddenly realise what is going on?*

⌘ Made actions or experiences:

> *Do you ever feel that your actions are controlled by somebody else?*
> *Are your feelings or your emotions not your own?*

Do you feel you are made to do things over which you have no control?

⌘ Somatic hallucinations:

Do you feel your body is being interfered with?
Have you had any strange physical experiences?
Have you experienced being influenced from outside yourself by powers like waves or rays?

Explores passivity phenomena   `A` `B` `C` `D` `E`

Factual content   `A` `B` `C` `D` `E`

Global score   `A` `B` `C` `D` `E`

22. Suicidal intent after an overdose

Introduces self and explains reason for the assessment.
Establishes rapport.
Shows empathy.

Introduction   `A` `B` `C` `D` `E`

Establishes rapport   `A` `B` `C` `D` `E`

Empathy   `A` `B` `C` `D` `E`

Listening skills   `A` `B` `C` `D` `E`

⌘ Establishes the following information about the overdose:

- how many tablets were taken
- what type of medication
- when was the overdose taken
- how was the medication obtained.

Elicits basic history   `A` `B` `C` `D` `E`

⌘ Establishes details of the circumstances:

- where was the patient when he took the overdose
- did he take any precautions to prevent being found?
- did he expect anybody to find him?
- how and by whom was he discovered?
- how did he reach hospital?

Explores circumstances | A | | B | | C | | D | | E | |

Precaution taken | A | | B | | C | | D | | E | |

⌘ Tries to establish information about the seriousness of the attempt:

- how long had the overdose been planned?
- did he mention his intentions to anyone?
- what did he expect would happen?
- did he expect to die?
- what about if he was found and received medical attention?
- did he leave a suicide note?

Degree of planning | A | | B | | C | | D | | E | |

Precautions taken | A | | B | | C | | D | | E | |

⌘ Tries to find out about other element s that might have played a role, such as

- physical illness
- mood symptoms
- signs of psychosis
- personality difficulties
- substance misuse.

Explores comorbid symptoms | A | | B | | C | | D | | E | |

⌘ Forms an opinion about seriousness, taking into consideration:

- physical illness
- divorce
- planned
- taken while alone
- intended to die
- suicide note.

⌘ Mentions need for further assessment, treatment and support in view of high degree of intent.

Summarization | A | | B | | C | | D | | E | |

Ending | A | | B | | C | | D | | E | |

23. Personality

Introduces self and explains the reason for the assessment.
Establishes rapport.
Shows empathy.
Asks open as well as closed questions.

Listening skills	A	B	C	D	E

Question framing	A	B	C	D	E

Verbal facilitation	A	B	C	D	E

⌘ Explores relationships:

> *Are you currently in a relationship?*
> *How long have you been together?*
> *How is your relationship at the moment?* **or** *How do you get on?*
> *Do you have any children?*
> *Have you had any other relationships?*
> *Do you have any other friends?*
> *How do you usually get on with other people?*
> *Is it important for you to be with somebody?*

⌘ Work:

> *How long have you been in your current job?*
> *Have you had any other jobs?*
> *Have you been out of work for any period of time? Can you tell me what happened?*

Assessment of work and relationships	A	B	C	D	E

⌘ Assesses prevailing mood:

> *How has your mood been lately?* **or** *What's your mood like generally?*
> *Are you always anxious or worried?*
> *Is there anything you do to make yourself feel less anxious?*
> *Do you ever feel as if you are empty inside, as if you have no emotion?*
> *Do you have mood-swings?*
> *Do you still get pleasure out of activities you normally enjoy?*
> *Do you feel your life is worth living?*
> *How often do you have thoughts of ending your life or harming yourself?*
> *Have you harmed yourself in any way, for example, by taking overdoses of medication or cutting yourself? How often have you done so?*

⌘ Assesses self-esteem:

> *How do you feel about yourself?*
> *How is your self-esteem?*
> *Do you retain your sense of self-worth and usefulness?*

⌘ Assesses coping strategies for, and capacity to deal with, stress.

⌘ Assesses strong religious convictions or other personal beliefs.

⌘ Assesses tolerance to frustration.

Mood and self-esteem | A | | B | | C | | D | | E | |

⌘ Substance misuse:

> *Do you currently use any illicit drugs or alcohol?*
> *What kinds of drugs have you used previously?*
> *How much do you use/drink in the average day/week?*

⌘ Forensic history:

> *Have you ever had trouble with the police or the criminal justice system?*
> *Do you have any prior convictions? Have you ever been imprisoned? Have*
> *you ever been under probation?*

Substance misuse and forensic history | A | | B | | C | | D | | E | |

⌘ Psychotic symptoms:

> *Do you hear peoples' voices when there is no one around?* **or** *Do you ever*
> *see or hear anything unusual that you can't explain?*
> *Do you ever feel that people are conspiring against you, or that they are*
> *plotting to harm you in some way?*

⌘ Also explores ideas of reference and other delusional beliefs in brief.

Psychotic symptoms | A | | B | | C | | D | | E | |

⌘ Personal history:

> *Did your parents work? What did they do?*
> *What was their relationship like?*
> *What was the atmosphere at home like? How did you get on with your*
> *parents?*
> *Did you have any brothers or sisters?*

> *From what you have been told, were there any problems in your early development? Did you walk and talk at the right times?*
> *What kind of an upbringing did you have?*
> *Did you have any problems at school? Were you bullied? Did you have any other problems in childhood, such as being abused physically or in any other way?*

Personal history | A | | B | | C | | D | | E | |

Global rating | A | | B | | C | | D | | E | |

24. Mini Mental State Examination (copyright 1983, Folstein MF Robins LN, Helzer JE, *Archives of General Psychiatry*, **40**(7): 812)

Establishes rapport, explains the purpose of the test and asks for consent to proceed.
Gives clear instructions.
Is reassuring and encouraging.
Is sensitive to patient's difficulties, and does not rush patient along.
States that questions vary in terms of difficulty.

Consent | A | | B | | C | | D | | E | |

Explanation | A | | B | | C | | D | | E | |

Question framing | A | | B | | C | | D | | E | |

Orientation in time

Maximum score of five points, one point each for year, season, day, date and month.
Asks additional questions, 'Can you tell me what season we're in?'

Orientation in place

Maximum score of five points, one each for country, county, city/town/village, building, floor/ward.
Asks for further clarification: 'What kind of building are we in?'

Orientation in time and place | A | | B | | C | | D | | E | |

Registration

- informs the patient that he/she would like to test his memory
- gives him three unrelated words and asks him to repeat these words
- takes about a second for each word

- prompts the patient to remember the three words, as they will be asked about them again
- gives one point for each word repeated the first time
- repeats the words until he has learned all three
- maximum score three points.

Attention

- asks the patient whether he can spell the word 'world'. Then asks if he can spell it backwards
- gives one point for each letter in the correct (reverse) order
- maximum score five points
- alternatively, asks the patient to subtract 7 from 100 and continue to do this; checks the answers 93, 86, 79, 72, 65 and gives a point for each correct answer maximum score five points.

Recall

- asks whether the patient can recall any of the three words he was asked to remember
- one point for each correct answer, maximum three points.

Registration, attention and recall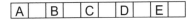

Naming

- shows the patient a watch and a pen and asks him what they are
- one point for each correct answer, maximum two points.

Repetition

- asks the patient to repeat the sentence: 'no ifs, ands or buts'
- allows only one attempt, one point if repeated correctly.

Three-stage command

- hands the patient a sheet of paper
- gives a clear instruction: 'Take this paper in your right hand, fold it in half and put it on the floor'
- one point for each correct action, maximum three points.

Naming, repetition, three-stage command ⌐A⌐ ⌐B⌐ ⌐C⌐ ⌐D⌐ ⌐E⌐

Reading

- writes the instruction 'CLOSE YOUR EYES' in large letters
- asks the patient to, 'read it and do what it says'

- one point if the patient closes his eyes.

Writing

- asks the patient to write a sentence, to be written spontaneously
- scores one point when the sentence makes sense and has a subject and a verb
- allow for errors in spelling and grammar.

Copying

- draws two intersecting pentagons (as below)
- asks the patient to copy the drawing exactly
- one point if the pentagons intersect correctly and the intersection has four angles.

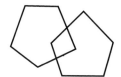

Reading, writing and copying	A	B	C	D	E
Summarization	A	B	C	D	E
Ending	A	B	C	D	E
Global rating	A	B	C	D	E

Section three:
Procedure skills

3.1

Instructions for candidates

---

25. Testing of arm and hand function

Test tone, power, sensation (apart from pain and temperature) and coordination in this patient's arm and hand.

26. Obtain consent and perform an ECG recording

You are asked by your consultant to perform an ECG recording on a patient that is due to commence an anti-psychotic medication. Your consultant wants your opinion on the corrected Q–T interval. Your patient (represented by this manikin) has been prepared for the procedure by the staff nurse on the ward. He is lying on a couch in your clinic room, stripped to the waist and with exposed ankles.

Record an ECG on this patient.

27. Alcohol dependence — physical examination

This fifty-four-year-old man, who has been drinking alcohol to excess for many years, has come to hospital this morning for detoxification from alcohol. He had his last drink at around 10.00 pm.

Physically examine this patient, with special attention to problems related to his alcohol abuse, and explain what you are doing.

28. Opiate dependence — physical examination

You are called to see a twenty-four-year-old lady with a long history of heroin abuse, who was admitted to hospital last night.

Physically examine this patient with special attention to problems related to her heroin abuse, and explain what you are doing.

29. Extra-pyramidal side-effects — physical examination

This fifty-year-old lady has noticed abnormal movement in her hands. She has been receiving a depot injection of flupenthixol for the last twelve years.

Physically examine this patient for extra-pyramidal side-effects.

30. Neuroleptic malignant syndrome

You are called to an acute admissions ward by nursing staff who are concerned about a thirty-year-old male patient. He has a long history of paranoid schizophrenia, and until recently was on a weekly fluphenazine depot injection. He was switched onto a haloperidol depot injection five days ago. Today he has been drowsy, uncommunicative, and is feverish.

Assess the patient for symptoms and signs of neuroleptic malignant syndrome (NMS). Assuming you have confirmed a diagnosis of NMS, explain to the patient what you are going to do next.

31. Serotonin syndrome

A thirty-five-year-old teacher has been attending your out-patient clinic for the last two years for treatment of her depression. At your last appointment you decided to switch her to a newer antidepressant, after tapering off her previous one (a monoamine oxidase inhibitor). Today, she has come to your clinic and says she has felt irritable lately, has been sweating profusely, and has had diarrhoea and abdominal pain for the last day.

Take a brief history and physically examine this patient for symptoms of serotonin syndrome.

32. Examination of cranial nerves (1)

Physically examine cranial nerves II to VII on this patient, except for testing of the corneal reflex, sense of taste, and fundoscopy.

33. Examination of cranial nerves (2)

Physically examine cranial nerves VIII to XII on this patient.

34. Fundoscopic examination of the eye

Examine the optic fundi of this patient (represented by a manikin) and describe any abnormal findings.

25. Testing of arm and hand function

The actor is advised to act as normal. This station involves the candidate physically examining you.

Please follow any instructions given to you by the candidate.

26. Obtain consent and perform an ECG recording

A manikin is provided for this station.

27. Alcohol dependence — physical examination

The actor is advised to act as normal. This station involves the candidate physically examining you.

Please follow any instructions given to you by the candidate.

28. Opiate dependence — physical examination

You are a twenty-four-year-old girl, who has been injecting herself four times a day with heroin for the last two years. You inject yourself mainly in the groin and neck. You snort cocaine on occasion. Your GP has recently told you that you have hepatitis C infection. One of the injection sites in the groin has become infected and is leaking pus.

29. Extra-pyramidal side effects — physical examination

You are fifty-year-old lady, with a long history of schizophrenia. Your doctors have tried many medications over the years, before settling on a two-weekly depot injection twelve years ago. A few weeks ago, you noticed funny movements in your hands. Your family have noticed grimacing movements around your mouth, which you are not aware of. At times, you have found it difficult to walk properly, as there is stiffness in your legs.

30. Neuroleptic malignant syndrome

You are a thirty-year-old man, who has been living in a nursing home for some years. You have been admitted to hospital so that your depot injection can be changed to a different one to see if this can better deal with the voices you hear. You had a test dose of the new injection about five days ago. Since yesterday, you have been feeling very unwell and dizzy. When the nurse called you for breakfast this morning, you could not remember where you were and you stayed in bed. You are feeling very hot and are sweating a lot. Your muscles feel tense.

31. Serotonin syndrome

You are a thirty-five-year-old school teacher, who has been attending the psychiatric out-patient clinic for the last two years. Your depression has improved but your doctor thinks you may do better on a newer antidepressant. You started it last week, but continued taking the old one despite his advice to stop it completely, because you were worried at not having enough antidepressant in your system. You have noticed that you have been having sweats lately, but thought this might be related to your periods. Your work colleagues have said that you have been irritable with them in the last week, and you have found yourself getting easily upset with some of the students. This morning, you had abdominal pains and diarrhoea. You remembered the doctor asking you to make an urgent appointment if you felt at all unwell and so requested one today.

32. Examination of cranial nerves (1)

The actor is advised to act as normal. This station involves the candidate physically examining you.

Please follow any instructions given to you by the candidate.

33. Examination of cranial nerves (2)

The actor is advised to act as normal. This station involves the candidate physically examining you.

Please follow any instructions given to you by the candidate.

34. Fundoscopic examination of the eye

A manikin is provided for this station.

3.3

Instructions for examiners

25. Testing of arm and hand function

Introduces self and explains purpose of the examination.
Gives clear instructions.
Is friendly and patient.

Consent

A	B	C	D	E

Explanation

A	B	C	D	E

Use of language

A	B	C	D	E

⌘ Tests muscle tone:

- moves elbow and wrist passively.

⌘ Tests muscle power:

- flexion and extension at the elbow
- flexion and extension at the wrist
- pronation of the fore-arm
- extension of the fingers
- hand grip
- adduction and abduction of thumb and fingers
- opposing thumb to base of the little finger.

Tone and power

A	B	C	D	E

⌘ Tests deep tendon reflexes:

- biceps
- triceps
- supinator.

Reflexes

A	B	C	D	E

⌘ Tests sensation

- light touch

- joint position sense
- finger recognition
- stereognosis.

Sensation | A | | B | | C | | D | | E | |

⌘ Tests coordination:

- finger – nose test
- alternating hand movements
- fine movements
- touching fingers with thumb
- writing.

Coordination | A | | B | | C | | D | | E | |

Interaction with patient | A | | B | | C | | D | | E | |

Global rating | A | | B | | C | | D | | E | |

26. Obtain consent and perform an ECG recording

As this station has a manikin representing the patient, some of the conversation may be addressed to the examiner. You may start by stating that a chaperone would usually be present for the procedure.

Introduces self and explains reason for examination:

> *This test is done to examine the electrical activity of your heart, by taking a tracing through these electrodes called 'leads'. The procedure is painless as the leads are simply placed across your chest on top of your skin. This is a diagram that shows you where I will place the electrodes.*
> *I will talk you through each step of the procedure.*

⌘ Reiterates the need to do the test prior to starting the new medication.

⌘ Reassures him that the procedure will be stopped if he is uncomfortable at any stage.

⌘ Explains the various steps of the procedure.

⌘ Asks for any questions the patient may have.

⌘ Obtains verbal consent to perform the test.

⌘ Explains each step again as it is performed.

Introduction | A | | B | | C | | D | | E | |

Explanation of procedure | A | | B | | C | | D | | E | |

Obtains verbal consent | A | | B | | C | | D | | E | |

⌘   Test procedure:

- attach the limb leads to all four limbs, using contact gel under each electrode
- ensure good contact with the skin
- positioning of chest leads:
  V1 — fourth intercostal space at right sternal border
  V2 — fourth intercostal space at left sternal border
  V3 — midway between leads V2 and V4
  V4 — fifth intercostal space in the midclavicular spaceV5 — anterior axillary line at the same horizontal level as lead V4
  V6 — mid-axillary line at the same horizontal level as leads V4 and V5.
- switch on the machine and make the recording. Once completed, dispose of the electrode pads and waste appropriately.

Procedure | A | | B | | C | | D | | E | |

Explanation of steps to patient | A | | B | | C | | D | | E | |

Positioning of leads | A | | B | | C | | D | | E | |

Ending | A | | B | | C | | D | | E | |

Global rating | A | | B | | C | | D | | E | |

27. Alcohol dependence — physical examination

Introduces self and explains the purpose of the examination.
Obtains verbal consent.
Gives clear instructions.
It may be useful to mention out aloud what you are looking for.

Introduction | A | | B | | C | | D | | E | |

Obtains consent | A | | B | | C | | D | | E | |

Explains findings at each step | A | | B | | C | | D | | E | |

⌘   Observes for signs of withdrawal:

- agitation, restlessness, anxiety

- tremor ('the shakes')
- autonomic nervous system hyperactivity, manifesting as sweating and raised temperature
- hypertension (particularly raised systolic pressure), tachycardia
- tachypnoea
- increased deep tendon reflexes.

Withdrawal symptoms   [A] [B] [C] [D] [E]

⌘ General examination:

- bruises, abrasions, scars suggestive of falls or violence
- facial redness, bilateral parotid enlargement
- spider naevi mainly on trunk, face and arms
- icterus and scratch marks
- signs of self neglect or immuno-deficiency, such as fungal infections
- muscle wasting
- gynaecomastia and testicular atrophy
- decreased body hair.

⌘ Examines hands for:

- palmar erythema
- clubbing
- nail changes
- nicotine stains or cigarette burns
- Dupuytren's contracture.

⌘ Examines the eyes for:

- icterus
- pallor
- nystagmus
- eye movements, in particular, lateral gaze palsy (abducens nerve).

Inspection   [A] [B] [C] [D] [E]

Appropriate instructions   [A] [B] [C] [D] [E]

⌘ Examines cardiovascular system for:

- tachycardia, hypertension
- arrhythmias — ventricular extrasystoles, (paroxysmal) atrial fibrillation
- congestive cardiac failure secondary to alcoholic cardiomyopathy
- peripheral oedema.

⌘ Examines respiratory system for:

- signs of congestive cardiac failure
- chest infection.

Examination of cardiovascular system |A| |B| |C| |D| |E|

⌘ Examines the abdomen using percussion and palpation for:

- hepatomegaly
- firm, nodular and small liver (cirrhosis)
- splenomegaly
- ascites
- caput medusae (dilated veins on the abdominal wall).

Examination of abdomen |A| |B| |C| |D| |E|

⌘ Performs a neurological examination, including:

- eye movements and nystagmus
- muscle tone and power
- peripheral sensation
- reflexes
- gait
- coordination.

Relevant neurological examination |A| |B| |C| |D| |E|

Ending |A| |B| |C| |D| |E|

Global rating |A| |B| |C| |D| |E|

28. Opiate dependence — physical examination

Introduces self and explains the purpose of the examination.
Obtains verbal consent.
Gives clear instructions.
It may be useful to mention out aloud what you are looking for.

Introduction |A| |B| |C| |D| |E|

Obtains consent |A| |B| |C| |D| |E|

Explains findings at each step |A| |B| |C| |D| |E|

⌘ With the patient standing, observes for signs of withdrawal:

- agitation, restlessness, anxiety, excessive yawning
- autonomic nervous system hyperactivity, manifesting as sweating and raised temperature, hypo- or hypertension, tachycardia
- dilated pupils, watery eyes, runny nose, goose flesh.

Obtain consent to do random blood glucose testing (hyperglycemia in withdrawals).

Withdrawal symptoms | A | B | C | D | E |

⌘ With the patient lying on a couch, general examination:

- bruises, abrasions, scars suggestive of falls or violence
- icterus and scratch marks
- splinter haemorrhages in nail beds
- signs of self-neglect or immuno-deficiency, such as fungal infections
- muscle wasting
- Roth's spots on fundoscopy of the eye.

General examination | A | B | C | D | E |

⌘ Examines for:

- injection site distribution
- abcesses or local inflammation
- evidence of recent use.

Inspection | A | B | C | D | E |

Appropriate instructions | A | B | C | D | E |

⌘ Examines cardiovascular system for:

- tachycardia, hypertension
- murmurs.

⌘ Examines respiratory system for:

- signs of congestive cardiac failure
- chest infection.

⌘ Examines the abdomen using percussion and palpation for:

- hepatomegaly
- splenomegaly.

⌘ Performs a neurological examination, including:

- muscle tone and power
- peripheral sensation
- reflexes
- gait and co-coordination.

Relevant systemic examination   A   B   C   D   E

Ending   A   B   C   D   E

Global rating   A   B   C   D   E

29. Extra-pyramidal side-effects — physical examination

Introduces self and explains the purpose of the examination.
Obtains verbal consent.
Gives clear instructions.
It may be useful to mention out aloud what you are looking for.

Introduction   A   B   C   D   E

Obtains consent   A   B   C   D   E

Explains findings at each step   A   B   C   D   E

⌘ General examination:

- observes the patient for obvious abnormal movements
- looks for dentures or braces
- determines the patient's level of distress
- examines arms for tremor.

Inspection   A   B   C   D   E

Appropriate instructions   A   B   C   D   E

⌘ Oral examination:

- observes the face and mouth, look for:
- looks for overt orofacial dyskinetic movements:
  - pouting
  - grimacing
- examines the tongue:
  - observe for repetitive, darting movements.

Orofacial movements   A   B   C   D   E

⌘ Performs a neurological examination, including:

- muscle tone, looking for rigidity
- pill rolling movements of the fingers
- reflexes
- gait and coordination.

Relevant neurological examination   A [ ] B [ ] C [ ] D [ ] E [ ]

Instructions to patient   A [ ] B [ ] C [ ] D [ ] E [ ]

Ending   A [ ] B [ ] C [ ] D [ ] E [ ]

Global rating   A [ ] B [ ] C [ ] D [ ] E [ ]

30. Neuroleptic malignant syndrome

Introduces self and explains the purpose of the examination.
Obtains verbal consent.
Gives clear instructions.
It may be useful to mention out aloud what you are looking for.
If there is an informant, confirms the details provided on the phone. Check for history of previous NMS, catatonia, known organic brain disorder, and ECT.
Also, ask if the patient has been ensuring hydration by drinking enough fluids.
Has the patient been agitated recently or needed restraint?

Introduction   A [ ] B [ ] C [ ] D [ ] E [ ]

Confirms history   A [ ] B [ ] C [ ] D [ ] E [ ]

Obtains consent   A [ ] B [ ] C [ ] D [ ] E [ ]

Explains findings at each step   A [ ] B [ ] C [ ] D [ ] E [ ]

⌘ General examination, look for:

- pallor
- unsteadiness of gait
- diaphoresis
- excessive salivation
- evidence of urinary incontinence.

⌘ Record his temperature, using instruments provided.

⌘ Ask the patient how he is feeling and explain in advance what you will be examining in broad terms. Then explain each step of the procedure:

I am going to examine you to find out how well you are physically. Could I start by asking you to put this thermometer under your tongue and hold it there for a little while?

Inspection

| A | B | C | D | E | |

Appropriate instructions

| A | B | C | D | E | |

⌘ Examines motor system, look for:

- generalised muscular hypertonicity (check both muscle tone, looking for the typical 'lead pipe' rigidity and deep tendon reflexes), which may also manifest as dyspnoea, and dysphagia.

⌘ Assesses mental state, look for:

- mutism, stupor and impaired consciousness. (The most useful way is to rate the patient's level of consciousness on the Glasgow Coma Scale and look for responsiveness to the external environment.)

⌘ Assesses autonomic signs:

- record his blood pressure (usually fluctating) and pulse rate (usually tachycardic).

Relevant physical examination

| A | B | C | D | E | |

⌘ Explains to the patient about the provisional diagnosis of NMS.

⌘ Explains how blood tests need to be done to confirm the diagnosis (this includes white cell count, Us and Es, LFTs, and Creatinine Kinase).

⌘ Discusses the initial management plan.

Explanation of diagnosis

| A | B | C | D | E | |

Reassurance

| A | B | C | D | E | |

Further management

| A | B | C | D | E | |

Ending

| A | B | C | D | E | |

Global rating

| A | B | C | D | E | |

31. Serotonin syndrome

Introduces self.
Reassures the patient that it was appropriate to seek help.

Introduction | A | | B | | C | | D | | E | |

Reassurance | A | | B | | C | | D | | E | |

Explains findings at each step | A | | B | | C | | D | | E | |

⌘ Talks about appropriateness of response to agreed plan.

⌘ Discusses exactly what has brought the patient to see you for an urgent appointment. Talk about the plan that was decided at the last appointment, and how the patient has put it into practice.

⌘ Examines the reasons why the patient did not follow the advice about discontinuing the previous antidepressant abruptly.

⌘ Explores the symptoms, particularly looking for onset, duration and progress of symptoms.

Relevant history | A | | B | | C | | D | | E | |

⌘ Explains to the patient that she will need to be examined to make it clear whether what she is experiencing is in any way related to the interaction of her antidepressants.

⌘ Obtains verbal consent for examination.

⌘ Gives clear instructions. It may be useful to mention out aloud what you are looking for.

⌘ Examines for:

- fever, tremor, confusion (test orientation to time, place, and person), level of consciousness (using the Glasgow Coma Scale). Observe for any overt manifestation of agitation or hypomania.

⌘ Specific examination:

- myoclonus, nystagmus, rigidity, cardiac arrythmias.

Obtains consent | A | | B | | C | | D | | E | |

Explains findings at each step | A | | B | | C | | D | | E | |

⌘ Explains to the patient about the provisional diagnosis that has been made.

> At this stage it is essential to use simple language. NMS can be described as a, 'rare but serious reaction to the new drug'. The key point is to reassure the patient that it has been found at an early stage and appropriate treatment can therefore be started immediately.

⌘ Discusses the initial steps in management.

⌘ You would be expected to mention the stopping of all serotonergic medication, including both of her antidepressants, and managing hyperpyrexia. Emphasise close liaison with your colleagues on the medical wards.

Explanation of diagnosis	A	B	C	D	E
Reassurance	A	B	C	D	E
Further management	A	B	C	D	E
Ending	A	B	C	D	E
Global rating	A	B	C	D	E

Given the suggested diagnosis, look for a picture that is consistent with Sternbach's (1991) diagnostic criteria for serotonin syndrome which consist of:

1. At least three of: agitation/restlessness, sweating, diarrhoea, fever, hyperreflexia, lack of co-ordination, mental state changes (confusion hypomania), myoclonus, shivering, and tremor.
2. Other causes, such as infection, metabolic, substance abuse or withdrawal ruled out.
3. No concurrent antipsychotic changes prior to symptom onset.

32. Examination of cranial nerves (1)

Introduces self.
Explains the purpose of the examination.
Gives appropriate and clear instructions.
Avoids jargon.

Consent	A	B	C	D	E
Explanation	A	B	C	D	E
Use of language	A	B	C	D	E

Cranial nerve II

* ❖ Tests visual acuity using a Snellen chart, from a distance of six meters.
* ❖ Examines visual fields for each eye separately, with the other eye covered.
* ❖ Compares the patient's visual field with that of the examiner.
* ❖ Gives appropriate instructions, eg. to focus on examiner's nose.
* ❖ Tests the four quadrants of the visual field.
* ❖ Brings in a target from the peripheral to central field of vision.

Vision | A | B | C | D | E |

Cranial nerves III, IV and VI

* ❖ Inspects the eye for ptosis and size of pupils.
* ❖ Tests pupillary reflexes, namely direct light reflex, consensual light reflex and reaction to accommodation.
* ❖ Tests eye movements in all directions.
* ❖ Enquires about double vision.

Eye movements and reflexes | A | B | C | D | E |

Cranial Nerve V

* ❖ Tests sensation comparing both sides of forehead, cheeks and jaw.
* ❖ Tests jaw muscles by palpating the masseters.
* ❖ Asks the patient to clench his teeth.
* ❖ Asks the patient to open his mouth and move his jaw sideways.

Facial sensation and jaw muscles | A | B | C | D | E |

Cranial nerve VII

* ❖ Asks the patient to frown.
* ❖ Asks the patient to shut his eyes tightly and attempts to open them.
* ❖ Asks the patient to show his teeth, and then blow up his cheeks, and finally asks him to whistle.

Facial muscles | A | B | C | D | E |

Reassurance | A | B | C | D | E |

Ending | A | B | C | D | E |

Global rating | A | B | C | D | E |

33. Examination of cranial nerves (2)

Explains the purpose of the examination.
Gives appropriate and clear instructions.
Is polite and gentle.
Avoids jargon.

Consent | A | | B | | C | | D | | E | |

Explanation | A | | B | | C | | D | | E | |

Use of language | A | | B | | C | | D | | E | |

Cranial nerve VIII

- ❖ Tests patients ability to hear whispering or rubbing fingers.
- ❖ Tests each ear separately, while the other ear is kept closed.
- ❖ Asks whether the patient hears any ringing, buzzing or hissing sounds without any stimulus.
- ❖ Holds a tuning fork on the patient's mastoid. When the patient doesn't hear it anymore, holds it 1 cm from the ear and checks whether the patient hears it again. If so, Rinne's test is positive, which indicates no hearing loss.
- ❖ Places the tuning fork in the midline of the skull.
- ❖ Checks whether the patient hears better on one side (Weber's test) — in conductive deafness the patient hears better on the affected side.
- ❖ Asks about vertigo and checks for nystagmus.

Hearing and balance | A | | B | | C | | D | | E | |

Cranial nerves IX and X

- ❖ Notes difficulty in speaking, in particular, hoarseness and nasal speech.
- ❖ Asks the patient to say 'aah' and inspects the palate and uvula.
- ❖ Asks the patient to swallow.

Cranial Nerve XI

- ❖ Asks the patient to shrug his shoulders (trapezius muscle).
- ❖ Asks the patient to rotate his head against resistance (sternomastoid muscle).

Cranial Nerve XII

- ❖ Asks the patient to open his mouth.
- ❖ Inspects the tongue for wasting or fasciculation.
- ❖ Asks the patient to push his tongue against the inside of his cheek.
- ❖ Asks the patient to stick out his tongue and lick his lips.

Mouth, tongue and throat | A | | B | | C | | D | | E | |

Examination skills | A | | B | | C | | D | | E | |

Ending | A | | B | | C | | D | | E | |

Global rating | A | | B | | C | | D | | E | |

34. Fundoscopic examination of the eye

Introduces self and explains the purpose of the examination.
Obtains verbal consent.
Gives clear instructions.
It may be useful to mention out aloud what you are looking for.

Introduction | A | | B | | C | | D | | E | |

Obtains consent | A | | B | | C | | D | | E | |

Explains findings at each step | A | | B | | C | | D | | E | |

⌘ General procedure:

- checks that the ophthalmoscope is working properly
- asks the patient to gaze into the distance and/or focus on an object straight ahead
- holds the patient's upper eyelid open against the orbit
- uses the right eye to inspect the patient's right eye, holding the ophthalmoscope in the right hand and the same for the left side
- gets close to the patient and approaches the eye at an angle of 30°.
- sets the focus at the '0' position and rotates the dial clockwise and anti-clockwise.

Setting up instrument | A | | B | | C | | D | | E | |

Approach technique | A | | B | | C | | D | | E | |

⌘ Examines the optic disc:

- notes its margin, cup and colour
- notes the vessels radiating from the centre of the disc
- follows the four major vessels into each quadrant.

⌘ Recognizes a normal fundus:

- the optic disc is a full moon-like circle
- the margin is well defined, but less clear on the nasal side
- the centre is paler than the rim.

⌘ Recognizes papilloedema:

- swelling of the optic disc with blurring of the margin and possible haemorrhages
- usually associated with raised intracranial pressure.

⌘ Recognizes hypertensive retinopathy:

- swelling of the optic disc, with flame-shaped haemorrhages and cotton wool spots.

⌘ Recognizes diabetic retinopathy:

- the retina shows tiny red dots (microaneurysms), blots (haemorrhages) and waxy looking exudates.

Technique	A	B	C	D	E
Normal eye	A	B	C	D	E
Abnormal eye	A	B	C	D	E
Summarizes findings	A	B	C	D	E
Global rating	A	B	C	D	E

Section four:
Communication skills

Instructions for candidates

35. Discuss laboratory results

Discuss the following laboratory results with your patient. He was admitted to hospital two days ago with alcohol-related problems. Your patient wants to know if his liver has been damaged by his drinking.

Na^+	138 mmol/L	
K^+	3.6 mmol/L	
Cl^-	98 mmol/L	
HCO^-_3	27.5 mmol/L	
Platelets	280×10^9/L	
MCV	108 fl	**H**
Urea	170 mmol/L	
Creatinine	110 umol/L	
Hb	13. 5 g/dl	
ALT	185 U/L	**H**
AST	153 U/L	**H**
GGT	270 U/L	**H**

36. Drug misuse in pregnancy

This nineteen-year-old lady, who is dependent on heroin, is six weeks pregnant. She injects heroin, shares needles, and has become pregnant after having unprotected sex. She wants advice on her drug use and continuing the pregnancy. She is also worried about being infected with HIV.

37. Information for out-patient ECT

This patient was recently discharged from your in-patient ward after successful treatment with electroconvulsive therapy. Your consultant wants you to discuss with him the option of receiving ECT as an out-patient.

38. Prognosis in schizophrenia

The mother of an eighteen-year-old man wants to talk to you. Her son was admitted to hospital for the first time three weeks ago. He has been told he has schizophrenia.

Discuss the illness and its prognosis with her.

39. Aetiology of a psychotic episode

The father of a newly-admitted patient wants to talk to you. His son, a twenty-seven-year-old man, with a two-year history of glue sniffing, was brought in to hospital detained under Section 2 of the Mental Health Act 1983, after stopping his antipsychotic medication, assaulting his father and making violent threats to his neighbours in response to persecutory delusions.

Explore the etiological factors in this case through discussion with his father. His father also wants some explanation about the causes for his son's current condition.

40. Starting a patient on clozapine

A fifty-five-year-old patient, with a diagnosis of chronic paranoid schizophrenia, who has been on various combinations of medication, including depots over the last twenty years without improvement in his functioning, has come to your out-patient clinic. On review of his notes, you decide that he would probably benefit from being on clozapine and you would like to discuss this with him.

Discuss the potential benefits and problems of clozapine including side-effects. Explain how you would commence him on this medication.

41. Clozapine reaction

A fifty-seven-year-old lady with treatment-resistant schizophrenia is currently on clozapine. Her brother, who is her main carer, phones you and tells you that she is concerned that the patient has been poorly in the last few days. She has had flu-like symptoms since yesterday, and this morning developed a fever. You ask the patient to come to hospital immediately.

Explain to the patient what will happen now.

42. Alzheimer's disease

This lady's eighty-year-old mother has been increasingly forgetful in recent months. Her GP has mentioned that she may be suffering from Alzheimer's disease. The daughter has arranged to see you to ask you some questions.

Discuss the illness, its treatment and prognosis with her

43. Dementia treatment

The husband of a seventy-eight-year-old woman has asked to see you. His wife has recently been diagnosed with Alzheimer's disease. She scored 24/30 on a recent Mini Mental State Examination. The husband has been told that it may be possible for his wife to be started on medication for Alzheimer's disease, but he first would like to find out some more information.

Discuss the treatment options available.

44. Starting a patient on lithium

Mr A is a twenty-six-year-old single man who was admitted to your ward three weeks ago with elated mood, pressure of speech, flight of ideas and grandiose beliefs. He has been treated with olanzapine 5 mg twice a day and has shown a partial response. In the ward round it has been decided to try treatment with lithium. Mr A has some questions and has asked to see you.

Discuss lithium treatment with him. Assuming he agrees, how would you start him on it?

45. Discussing ECT as a treatment option

This patient was admitted five weeks ago with severe depression. He has not responded to antidepressant medication, even at higher doses and his physical health is deteriorating rapidly. Your consultant wants you to discuss electroconvulsive therapy with him and obtain consent if possible.

35. Discuss laboratory results

You are a twenty-seven-year-old man. You have been drinking daily for the last ten years and are concerned that you may have done some damage to your liver. You have been taking vitamin pills but nothing else. You had blood tests done a week ago and are meeting with the psychiatrist to discuss the results.

36. Drug misuse in pregnancy

You are nineteen years old and dependent on heroin which you inject four times a day. You share your drug supply and equipment with your friends. You have found out that you are six weeks pregnant. Though this was unplanned, you would like to continue with it. You have come to talk to the psychiatrist about coming off heroin and continuing the pregnancy. You are worried about the risks of heroin to your unborn child. You are also concerned about whether you might be infected with HIV and any impact this might have on the pregnancy and delivery.

37. Information for out-patient ECT

You are a fifty-eight-year-old bachelor. You live alone and have had a long-standing depressive illness. You have been treated with electroconvulsive (shock) therapy on several occasions, as an in-patient. Although you have only recently been discharged from hospital after your latest course of treatments, you think that you may be relapsing into another episode of low mood. ECT has always worked for you and you are familiar with its benefits and side-effects. You have heard that some people have ECT as out-patients once a month and that it keeps them well.

38. Prognosis in schizophrenia

You are the mother of an eighteen-year-old man. Your son has been in hospital for three weeks. There has been a gradual deterioration in his personality and self-care over the last two years. In recent months, he has been talking about how people have been abusing him and threatening to kill him. He said he could hear them talking about him late at night. He thought that they were observing him through special sensors. He dropped out of college and has lost all his friends. He was spending all of his time in his room. On the day he was admitted, he stabbed his brother after the voices had told him to do so. He has now been told he has a diagnosis of schizophrenia.

Your own mother died in a mental hospital. She also had the same illness.

39. Aetiology of a psychotic episode

You are a forty-nine-year-old teacher, who has come to hospital following the admission of your son. He was brought into hospital after he punched you in the head, saying you were reading his thoughts, and threatened the neighbours saying that they would be next on his list as they were spying on him with cameras and had implanted a microphone in his tooth. You have been told by the social worker that your son will be detained in hospital under a Section of the Mental Health Act for up to twenty-eight days. You had noticed that he was becoming more withdrawn in recent weeks, and you had found half-full tablet strips and some empty glue tubes in a corner of his room. You also know that some of his friends have drug habits, but you are not sure if your son uses anything. You have asked to meet with his doctor, as you want to know what has caused all of this, and especially whether you yourself caused this in some way.

40. Starting a patient on clozapine

You are a fifty-five-year-old man, who lives in a residential home. You have been hearing voices for most of your adult life, and have received treatment with many different combinations of medication, although they have never fully taken away the voices. At the moment, you are on a combination of a weekly injection and tablets. You have come for your three-monthly review at the out-patient clinic. Your psychiatrist wants to discuss a new medication with you. You have some questions for your psychiatrist about the benefits and problems of the new tablets.

41. Clozapine reaction

You are a fifty-seven-year-old lady with schizophrenia, who lives with your elderly brother. You have been treated with clozapine for a few years, and have been having blood tests every month. You have had a cough and sore throat since yesterday and this morning felt feverish. The psychiatrist told your brother to bring you to hospital immediately, but you do not know what the fuss is all about.

42. Alzheimer's disease

You are a fifty-year-old woman who works as a legal secretary. Your mother is eighty years old and has been living on her own since your father died of a heart-attack six years ago. She used to work as a primary school teacher and always has been very independent. Lately, however, she seems to be struggling; she always seems in a muddle, keeps repeating herself and often asks what day it is. You have spoken to her GP, who suspects that she is suffering from Alzheimer's disease. You are keen to get some more information about your mother's condition and would like to know more. You also have specific questions about how to cope with difficult behaviour and what you can expect for the future.

43. Dementia treatment

You are an eighty-year-old man. Your wife, who is seventy-eight, has become quite muddled lately. Your GP strongly suspects that she is suffering from Alzheimer's disease. He did a test which showed that her memory was not very good. You have been told that it may be worth finding out whether it would be possible for her to be treated with one of the new drugs for Alzheimer's. You had a look on the internet but found the information rather confusing. You are keen to get some more information about the treatment and would like to know more

44. Starting a patient on lithium

You are a twenty-six-year-old single man, who was admitted to the psychiatric ward three days ago. At the time your mood was very elated, you felt full of energy, and could not sit still. Your thoughts were racing and you were always rushing around. Initially, you were treated with olanzapine tablets once a day and you feel that there has been a gradual levelling out of your mood. At today's ward round, it was suggested that you be started on lithium. You would like to know more about lithium before you can agree to take it.

45. Discussing ECT as a treatment option

You are a fifty-four-year-old man, who has suffered from bouts of depression for a long time. You have been on various antidepressants in the past. You have now been in hospital — on this occasion, for five weeks. You have hardly been eating or drinking and the nurses are noting down your food and fluid intake. You are convinced that your life is not worth living and want to die. The only thing keeping you here is your concerns for your wife. This morning, in the ward round, it was suggested that you should consider having electroconvulsive therapy. All you know about it is from what you have seen in the movies, and what some of the other patients have said about it. Your doctor promised to talk to you about it outside the meeting.

35. Discuss laboratory results

Introduces self and explains reasons for meeting.
Enquires about what patient knows about the effects of drinking on the body.
Listens to patient and answers any queries.
Briefly asks about his current treatment.

Introduction   A   B   C   D   E

Listening skills   A   B   C   D   E

Ascertains patient's previous knowledge A   B   C   D   E

⌘ First shows the patient the results:

   • explains the different sections within the results
   • expands on the liver function tests
   • explains which the liver enzymes are, and their functions
   • explains the relevance of elevated levels
   • reassures the patient of the reversibility of the abnormal results
   • explains the diagnostic and therapeutic uses of testing for liver enzymes.

⌘ Expands on the haematology section:

   • explains what corpuscular volume is
   • explains its significance
   • discusses the probable causes for the abnormal results.

⌘ Reassures the patient that there is no need to panic about the results.

⌘ Explains that the results can be used to monitor the effects of treatment/interventions.

⌘ Checks with the patient about how much he has understood.

⌘ Asks for any further questions.

⌘ Restates the core of the information.

Use of language
A | B | C | D | E

Explanation
A | B | C | D | E

Factual content
A | B | C | D | E

Addresses questions and concerns
A | B | C | D | E

Summarization
A | B | C | D | E

Ending
A | B | C | D | E

Global rating
A | B | C | D | E

36. Drug misuse in pregnancy

Introduces self.
Explains reason for the interview.
Establishes rapport.
Finds out what patient wants out of the interview.
Uses a mixture of open and closed questions.

Introduction
A | B | C | D | E

Use of language
A | B | C | D | E

Establishes rapport
A | B | C | D | E

Establishes agenda
A | B | C | D | E

⌘ Initial discussion of the current drug use, such as type, amount and frequency of use.

⌘ Systematically looks at various scenarios:

- addresses problems with sudden discontinuation, such as abortion, still birth
- addresses consequences of continuation of current use, such as possible foetal anomalies.

⌘ Enquires as to what patient would like to do about her drug problem.

⌘ If she is adamant to continue using heroin, suggest referral to local drugs team.

⌘ Explores harm minimisation strategies, such as avoiding sharing needles, local needle exchanges and potential risk of harm to others and self from further infections.

⌘ Explains about pre- and post-test counselling for HIV and how the GUM clinic locally will help. Explains that all deliveries of those with HIV involve close liaison between the drugs team and the obstetrics team.

⌘ Mentions the likelihood that the neonate can have withdrawal symptoms at birth, and explains how they would be managed.

Discusses main options | A | B | C | D | E |

Examines each option in detail | A | B | C | D | E |

Mentions close liaison | A | B | C | D | E |

⌘ If she would like to come off the heroin before the birth, then discusses the various options available.

⌘ Explains about the best month for the drug to be withdrawn and the close liaison required with her obstetric team to monitor foetal safety.

⌘ Negotiates a clear management plan for subsequent visits and explores the support available to her.

⌘ Asks patient if she has any questions.

⌘ Offers contact numbers of relevant agencies and suitable information leaflets.

Discusses further management | A | B | C | D | E |

Addresses questions and concerns | A | B | C | D | E |

Factual knowledge | A | B | C | D | E |

Summarization | A | B | C | D | E |

Ending | A | B | C | D | E |

Global rating | A | B | C | D | E |

37. Information for out-patient ECT

Introduces self.
Explains reason for the interview.
Establishes rapport.

Introduction ⬜A⬜ ⬜B⬜ ⬜C⬜ ⬜D⬜ ⬜E⬜

Use of language ⬜A⬜ ⬜B⬜ ⬜C⬜ ⬜D⬜ ⬜E⬜

Establishes rapport ⬜A⬜ ⬜B⬜ ⬜C⬜ ⬜D⬜ ⬜E⬜

⌘ Explores patient's knowledge of ECT.

⌘ Briefly explains about the actual procedure:

- mentions the expected benefits
- discusses the potential side-effects
- mentions the precautions taken to deal with side-effects
- explains about general anaesthesia:
    explains about anaesthetic complications
    explains the need to fast from midnight on the previous day
- explains the importance of not taking any anticonvulsant, sedative or antidepressant medication until after the treatment
- explains precautions about driving
- explains advice to avoid travelling alone after treatment
- explains that he may have to spend the rest of the day at the local day centre, if he cannot ensure that someone will be able keep an eye on him.

Explores previous knowledge ⬜A⬜ ⬜B⬜ ⬜C⬜ ⬜D⬜ ⬜E⬜

Explanation of procedure ⬜A⬜ ⬜B⬜ ⬜C⬜ ⬜D⬜ ⬜E⬜

Discusses benefits and side-effects ⬜A⬜ ⬜B⬜ ⬜C⬜ ⬜D⬜ ⬜E⬜

Discusses specific precautions for out-patient ECT ⬜A⬜ ⬜B⬜ ⬜C⬜ ⬜D⬜ ⬜E⬜

⌘ Offer leaflets for further information.

⌘ Asks if patient has any questions and tries to answer them.

38. Prognosis in schizophrenia

Introduces self and explains reason for the interview.
Confirms that permission has been granted by the patient to discuss his illness, treatment and prognosis.
Establishes rapport.
Asks about previous knowledge of the illness.

Introduction   A   B   C   D   E

Use of language   A   B   C   D   E

Establishes rapport   A   B   C   D   E

⌘ Explains the prognostic factors associated with schizophrenia:

- discusses the importance of age of onset
- pre-morbid functioning
- duration of untreated illness
- pattern of onset, ie. whether sudden or insidious
- relevance of being male.

⌘ Explores family history of schizophrenia and explains its significance.

⌘ Reiterates importance of compliance with medication.

⌘ Mentions other factors with indirect links such as social isolation.

Explores relevant prognostic factors   A   B   C   D   E

Emphasis on positives   A   B   C   D   E

Addresses carer's concerns   A   B   C   D   E

Factual knowledge   A   B   C   D   E

Ending   A   B   C   D   E

Global rating   A   B   C   D   E

39. Aetiology of a psychotic episode

Introduces self and explains reasons for meeting.
Confirms that permission has been granted by the patient to discuss his illness:

> *Hello, Mr Roberts, I am Dr Marks. I understand you wanted to speak to me about your son, Tom. I have already asked him for permission to talk to you, in view of his right to confidentiality. There are a few bits of information that we hope you will be able to help us with. We can then perhaps look at what might have contributed to his being admitted here today.*

Establishes rapport.
Asks about previous knowledge of the illness.

Introduction | A | B | C | D | E |

Use of language | A | B | C | D | E |

Establishes rapport | A | B | C | D | E |

Explores prior knowledge | A | B | C | D | E |

⌘ Briefly discusses the presenting symptoms:

> *As you know, we think he may have been responding to persecutory beliefs when he attacked you and threatened the neighbours. These kind of fixed, unusual beliefs, which we call delusions, as well as hearing or seeing things that aren't there, which we call hallucinations, are together known as psychotic symptoms. They can, in some cases, occur as the result of mental illnesses like schizophrenia, and severe depression; physical illnesses, such as some forms of epilepsy; or even illicit drug use, such as heavy cocaine or amphetamine use.*

Mentions psychosis | A | B | C | D | E |

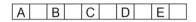

⌘ Explores aetiology in relation to differential diagnoses:

> *Has Tom ever had any form of mental illness? Has he ever received any treatment for this, and if so, what kind of treatment was it? Did he ever have to take a regular injection? Was this from his GP or has he been in contact with psychiatric services? Has he ever been admitted to a psychiatric hospital or day unit or has he attended an out-patient clinic? Does he have an allocated community psychiatric nurse or a social worker? Has he been taking his medication lately? Did he say he was happy to take his medication?*
>
> *I believe you found some empty glue tubes at home. Do you know if he regularly sniffs glue? Do you know if he uses any illicit drugs? Has he used*

any in the past? Has he ever injected drugs? Has he ever sought any help for his drug problem?

What about his physical health? Has he ever suffered from any serious physical illness, like diabetes or high blood pressure? Does he suffer from epilepsy? What type is it? Is he on medication for this? Does his GP or a specialist see him for this?

In the last few weeks, were you aware of any change in his behaviour? Has he been under any recent stress, or has he been worrying a lot lately? Has he had any major life events occur in his life lately, such as the death of someone close to him, or the loss of a job? Has there been any problem in any of his relationships with others?

History |A| |B| |C| |D| |E| |

Explores relevant aetiological factors |A| |B| |C| |D| |E| |

⌘ Discusses the current presentation and what will happen next

Perhaps we can now discuss what is going to happen next. As the social worker explained to you, Tom is now detained under Section 2 of the Mental Health Act, which allows his detention for up to twenty-eight days. This will allow him to be observed in hospital for further evidence of mental illness, and treatment as necessary. The leaflet you were given explains both his and your right of appealing against the detention. While he is here we will also do some investigations; including, blood tests, urine screening, an EEG (which is a recording of his brain's activity) and a scan of his head to rule out a physical cause like a tumour. At this stage, I must reassure you that these are routine investigations for someone presenting to us like your son.

Is there anything you would like to ask me at this stage?

Information on detention |A| |B| |C| |D| |E| |

Investigations |A| |B| |C| |D| |E| |

Addresses questions and concerns |A| |B| |C| |D| |E| |

Explains further management |A| |B| |C| |D| |E| |

Ending |A| |B| |C| |D| |E| |

Global rating |A| |B| |C| |D| |E| |

40. Starting a patient on clozapine

Introduces self and explains reason for the interview.
Establishes rapport.
Explains that in addition to reviewing how he has been since last seen, his medication is to be discussed in greater detail.

Introduction | A | B | C | D | E |

Use of language | A | B | C | D | E |

Establishes rapport | A | B | C | D | E |

Establishes agenda | A | B | C | D | E |

⌘ Reviews the patient's history, preferably asking for clarification or further information:

> *Having read through your medical notes, I wanted to clarify some of the important bits of information that I picked up on. Would it be correct to say that, since your first hospital admission when you were thirty-five years old, you have continued to hear voices more or less continuously? I had a look at all of the medications that you have had over the years. Which one do you think helped you the most? In what way do you feel it helped you? Why was it stopped? Are you still on it? Does/did it help to bring your voices under control? What kind of side-effects did you have on it?*

Overview of illness | A | B | C | D | E |

Confirms diagnosis | A | B | C | D | E |

Usefulness of medication | A | B | C | D | E |

⌘ Introduces clozapine, briefly mentioning the positive effects first:

> *I wanted to talk to you today about a drug that you haven't had before, although it belongs to the same group of drugs that you are currently on. It's called clozapine. Psychiatrists use it to help patients who have not responded to two or more drugs, what we call 'treatment-resistant schizophrenia'. Would you like me to tell you more? I will give you a leaflet with all of this information at the end of this meeting to take home and read.*
>
> *Clozapine is said to be particularly helpful for problems like being socially withdrawn, not communicating much, and having difficulty motivating yourself to do things. It can also help with certain side-effects of the usual drugs, like serious movement disorders.*

⌘ Mentions the relevant side-effects and precautions taken to minimise them:

Although it has so many good effects, it does have side-effects, some of which are less harmful, like drowsiness and constipation; some which are troublesome like weight gain, constipation and excessive salivation; and others that can be fatal like affecting your heart and bone marrow. We are fortunate that many of these side-effects are treatable. We try to manage weight gain by closely watching your diet and increasing your exercise levels, but this only helps with some of the weight gain. Other side-effects, like when it causes the bone marrow to produce fewer white blood cells, occur only rarely and need treatment on a medical ward. But because they can be serious, we try to catch them as soon as they occur, by checking your blood often. Initially, the blood tests are done every week for eighteen weeks, then every two weeks till a year is over and, thereafter, once a month for however long you are on it.

The main point is that once you are started on the drug, for which we need to admit you briefly in hospital, we will take every precaution to ensure your safety. If the blood results come back to us and are worrying in any way, we would contact you immediately, and call you in for a quick check-up. There are symptoms that you yourself could look out for that might help us pick up any problems before they become too serious. For example, if you have flu-like complaints such as fever or sore throat or you think you have an infection, you should have a blood test done here immediately. If you had any physical problem and were worried, you could always phone us for help or just come to see us.

Introduction to drug

| A | B | C | D | E |

Discussion on benefits and adverse effects

| A | B | C | D | E |

Precautions taken

| A | B | C | D | E |

Once you have read through the leaflet at home, let your CPN know what you think. He can answer any questions you have and discuss any particular concerns you may have. If you agree to take the drug, I would then have to send some of your details to register you with the agency set up by the drug company that makes clozapine. They would then send me a pack for your first blood test, so that they will have clear baseline values for how well your bone marrow, kidneys, liver and thyroid are functioning and your blood sugar and fat levels, before starting clozapine. I would then physically examine you, check your blood pressure and weigh you. I would also arrange for you to have an ECG, which is a tracing of the electrical activity of the heart, and an EEG which is a tracing of the electrical activity of your brain. Both of these tests are painless and take no more than half an hour. I will give you leaflets that explain them in more detail. We will only start you on the drug if it is safe to do so beforehand. Any questions?

Initiating treatment	A	B	C	D	E
Investigations	A	B	C	D	E
Addresses questions and concerns	A	B	C	D	E
Ending	A	B	C	D	E
Global rating	A	B	C	D	E

41. Clozapine reaction

Introduces self and explains urgency of the situation. Asks for permission to speak to her brother at the same time.

This is a case where you need to combine quick action with minimal distress to the patient. You could explain why you asked the patient to come to hospital so soon:

> *Hello, Ms Dalton. I am sorry I had to call you into hospital today. When your brother phoned me this morning, I was a bit concerned about how he said you were and asked him to bring you here just to make sure that we have nothing to worry about. I am going to ask you a few questions about your recent physical health and we will then need to do a blood test to make sure that you are safe to continue on clozapine.*

Introduction	A	B	C	D	E
Confidentiality	A	B	C	D	E
Establishes rapport	A	B	C	D	E
Establishes agenda	A	B	C	D	E

⌘ Explains in some detail why the patient had to be brought to hospital:

> *You may recall that when we first started you on clozapine, we said that there was a small chance that some patients might develop a serious side-effect to it. The side-effect is that it can affect your body by making fewer white blood cells, which can make you less able to fight off infections. The only way we can confirm if it is affecting you in this way is to do a blood test whenever you have symptoms of the flu.*

⌘ Rules out potential sources of infection/flu:

> *Do you remember the last time you were seen in the out-patient clinic we talked about how you need to watch for infections or the flu? Have you had anything like that in the last few days?*

I understand you were feeling feverish this morning. Would you mind if I check your temperature with this instrument?

Have you had any other signs that you might have an infection like a burning pain when passing water, or areas on your body where the skin is reddish and hot to touch?

Reasons for recall

A	B	C	D	E

Relevant history

A	B	C	D	E

⌘ Explains what will happen next:

First, I'll collect the sample of blood from you, and send it off to be analysed urgently. There are two different approaches that we will then take, depending on the results of the blood test. If it shows that your white blood cell count is low, I would then call my medical colleagues to discuss what should be done next. If it is particularly low, you would stop taking the clozapine and expect to be admitted to a medical ward for a while to allow your body to recover and to keep you safe from further infection. If it were not too low we would stop the clozapine and monitor your progress by doing further blood tests while you are an in-patient on one of our wards. Although this side-effect is usually reversible, we would need to make sure of your safety while we waited for it to improve. If, on the other hand, the result was normal, I would make a note of it in your medical records and we can then continue prescribing the clozapine for you. Your blood tests would continue as usual. Do you have any questions?

⌘ At this stage you would proceed with collecting a sample of blood for an urgent Full Blood Count. Explain the procedure to the patient and ask for permission.

Further management

A	B	C	D	E

Addresses concerns

A	B	C	D	E

Ending

A	B	C	D	E

Global rating

A	B	C	D	E

42. Alzheimer's disease

Introduces self and clarifies the reasons for the interview.
Establishes rapport.
Explores what the daughter already knows.
Gives a clear explanation, without using jargon.

Listening skills | A | | B | | C | | D | | E | |

Communication | A | | B | | C | | D | | E | |

Use of language | A | | B | | C | | D | | E | |

⌘ Points out the following characteristics:

- it is a type of dementia
- it is the most common form
- there are certain abnormalities in the brain
- nerve cells show signs of damage
- there is a decrease in brain tissue
- it presents as slow progressive decline in functioning
- often starts with memory problems and disorientation
- others areas of functioning are affected as well, such as language, self-care, practical skills and mood.

Explanation of nature | A | | B | | C | | D | | E | |

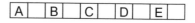

⌘ Explains that there is not one single known cause, but that there are some well recognized risk factors like:

- increasing age, especially over the age of seventy
- it can, although not always, run in certain families
- past history of head injury
- it is common in Down's syndrome
- possible role of common viral infections
- possible influence of poor academic achievement.

Etiology and risk factors | A | | B | | C | | D | | E | |

Overall knowledge | A | | B | | C | | D | | E | |

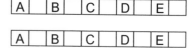

⌘ Explains that patients can sometimes be difficult to manage:

- ask the same questions over and over again
- make frequent phone-calls
- have difficulty looking after themselves
- do not eat regularly
- become anxious or depressed
- become restless
- wander out of the house and may get lost
- fail to recognize familiar faces
- become aggressive
- behave inappropriately
- are vulnerable to being taken advantage of and to being abused.

Behavioural difficulties | A | B | C | D | E |

⌘ Mentions that people tend to go downhill slowly over years. They become increasingly dependent and in the end may well need high levels of care. Suggests other possibilities for support:

- home care
- possibility of day-care, such as in a day centre
- community psychiatric nurse support
- voluntary organisations
- Alzheimer's society
- respite care
- residential or nursing-home care.

⌘ Examines medication briefly:

- medication like anti-Alzheimer's drugs
- other types of medication like calming drugs or anti-depressants.

Checks carer's concerns | A | B | C | D | E |

Advice about management | A | B | C | D | E |

Ending | A | B | C | D | E |

Global rating | A | B | C | D | E |

43. Dementia treatment

Introduces him/herself.
Establishes rapport.
Explores what the husband knows already.
Gives a clear explanation, without using jargon.

Listening skills | A | B | C | D | E |

Explanation | A | B | C | D | E |

Use of language | A | B | C | D | E |

⌘ Explains that recently new forms of treatment have become available and points out the following characteristics:

- it is only used in mild to moderate Alzheimer's disease
- it works by increasing a chemical substance in the brain, called acetylcholine

- the levels of acetylcholine in the brain are low in dementia
- drugs are called cholinesterase-inhibitors (not anti-cholinesterase-inhibitors, examples are donepezil [Aricept], galantamine [Reminyl], rivastigmine [Exelon])
- it does not cure the illness, but can slow down the decline
- it does not work in everyone
- you can only find out if it works, by trying it out on the patient.

General information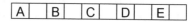

⌘ Gives appropriate information about side-effects, for example:

- the medication will be started at a low dose and can be increased if tolerated well
- common side-effects are nausea, diarrhoea, muscle cramps and sleeplessness
- people who have asthma, heart disease or stomach problems like ulcers may not be able to take it.

Cautions and side-effects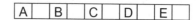

⌘ Points out National Institute of Clinical Excellence (NICE) guidelines, for example:

- there are certain guidelines (NICE) issued by the Department of Health
- it has to be started by a psychiatrist with special knowledge of dementia
- response to treatment will be monitored by doing tests, like the MMSE
- it can only be continued when there is a clear benefit
- repeating the MMSE does help to see if the treatment is effective
- if there is no benefit the treatment will have to be stopped
- when the score on the MMSE drops below 12 the treatment has to be stopped
- follow-up will be arranged every few months, eg. in a memory-clinic
- because people can be forgetful they need a carer to give them the medication.

NICE guidelines $\boxed{A}$ $\boxed{B}$ $\boxed{C}$ $\boxed{D}$ $\boxed{E}$

⌘ Gives further advice, for example:

- stimulate her mentally
- avoid unreasonable demands
- healthy diet, physical activity
- offer pleasurable activities
- possibility of day-care, eg. in a day centre
- carer support groups
- home-care
- CPN support
- voluntary organisations

- Alzheimer's society
- respite care.

Additional general advice ⬚A⬚ ⬚B⬚ ⬚C⬚ ⬚D⬚ ⬚E⬚

Summarization ⬚A⬚ ⬚B⬚ ⬚C⬚ ⬚D⬚ ⬚E⬚

Check carer's concerns ⬚A⬚ ⬚B⬚ ⬚C⬚ ⬚D⬚ ⬚E⬚

Ending ⬚A⬚ ⬚B⬚ ⬚C⬚ ⬚D⬚ ⬚E⬚

Global rating ⬚A⬚ ⬚B⬚ ⬚C⬚ ⬚D⬚ ⬚E⬚

44. Starting a patient on lithium

Establishes rapport.
Is polite and empathic.
Does not use jargon.
Is sensitive to patient's concerns.

Listening skills ⬚A⬚ ⬚B⬚ ⬚C⬚ ⬚D⬚ ⬚E⬚

Verbal facilitation ⬚A⬚ ⬚B⬚ ⬚C⬚ ⬚D⬚ ⬚E⬚

Use of language ⬚A⬚ ⬚B⬚ ⬚C⬚ ⬚D⬚ ⬚E⬚

⌘ Addresses indications for lithium:

- elated mood
- lack of sleep
- impulsive behaviour
- grandiose ideas
- overspending.

⌘ Explains that lithium is a mood stabiliser, which has been shown to be effective in treatment for mania and in prevention of relapse in bipolar disorder.

Factual content ⬚A⬚ ⬚B⬚ ⬚C⬚ ⬚D⬚ ⬚E⬚

⌘ Explains side-effects, for example:

- gastro-intestinal disturbances and weight gain
- fine tremor, fatigue and drowsiness
- polydipsia and polyuria
- dry mouth and metallic taste
- acne.

Side-effects | A | | B | | C | | D | | E | |

⌘ Explains:

- that he needs a blood test to check renal and thyroid function
- that once lithium has been started the dose will be adjusted until the serum-lithium concentration is within the therapeutic range
- that lithium levels, renal and thyroid functions will continue to be monitored every three months
- that there is a chance of developing hypothyroidism
- that toxic levels can lead to GI or CNS disturbances, and explains what
- that lithium levels can be affected by diarrhoea, vomiting, renal impairment and drug interactions.

Summarization | A | | B | | C | | D | | E | |

Addresses patient's concerns | A | | B | | C | | D | | E | |

Ending | A | | B | | C | | D | | E | |

Global rating | A | | B | | C | | D | | E | |

45. Discussing ECT as a treatment option

Introduces self and explains reason for the interview.
Confirms that permission has been granted by the patient to discuss his illness, treatment and prognosis.
Establishes rapport.
Asks about previous knowledge of the procedure.

Introduction | A | | B | | C | | D | | E | |

Use of language | A | | B | | C | | D | | E | |

Establishes rapport | A | | B | | C | | D | | E | |

⌘ Explains what ECT is and how it is thought to work:

During ECT a small amount of current is sent to the brain. This current is believed to activate various areas of brain concerning mood, sleep, appetite, and thinking centers. The current is believed to cause a change in the chemical balance bringing them to normal. This may help you to recover from your illness.

⌘ Expands on the use and types of ECT.

⌘ Explains the indications of ECT.

⌘ Explains the procedure:

> *You will need to wear loose clothes, remove jewellery, and dentures. Treatment will take place in a separate room. It will only take a few minutes, and nursing and medical staff will be with you throughout. An anaesthetist will give you an injection to make you sleep. Your muscles will relax completely and you will be given oxygen while you are asleep. Once you are fully asleep, a small electric current will be passed across your head using a machine. This causes you to have a fit, which, because you are asleep, you will not feel or remember. We will only observe you moving a little because of the relaxant given along with the anaesthetic. When you wake up you will be back in the waiting area.*

⌘ Explains other important details:

- the duration of treatment being a course of several treatments, usually between six to twelve, which are administered two to three times a week.
- the patient may need more than one course, but response to each course will be fully assessed
- the need to fast after mid-night from the previous day
- immediate side-effects after ECT such as headaches and confusion
- limitations of ECT, that it is another treatment for depression and will not cure marital or other problems
- the short-term memory problems after ECT must be mentioned, as well as the relative lack of evidence of longer term effects
- the 1 in 50,000 risk of death under general anaesthetic should be mentioned
- the patient should be reassured that consent will be taken at the start of the treatment course, but that he can choose to withdraw consent at any time.

As there is usually so much information being given at this time, it is usual to give the patient information leaflets, and encourage questions. Consent is usually obtained at a second or subsequent visit.

Explanation	A	B	C	D	E

Summarization	A	B	C	D	E

Addresses patient's concerns	A	B	C	D	E

Ending	A	B	C	D	E

Global rating	A	B	C	D	E

Useful resources

British National Formulary 45 (2003) *British National Formulary 45*. British Medical
  Association and the Royal Pharmaceutical Society of Great Britain, London
Cohen R (2000) *The Presentations of Clinical Psychiatry*. Quay Books, MA Healthcare
  Limited, Salisbury
Gelder M, Mayou R, Cowen P (2001) *Shorter Oxford Textbook of Psychiatry*. 4th edn. Oxford
  University Press, Oxford
Hodges JR (1993) *Cognitive Assessment for Clinicians*. Oxford University Press, Oxford
Jacoby R, Oppenheimer C (2002) *Psychiatry in the Elderly*. Oxford University Press, Oxford
Longmore JM, Longmore M, Wilkinson I, Torok E, eds (2001) *Oxford Handbook of Clinical
  Medicine*. 5th edn. Oxford University Press, Oxford
Munro JF, Campbell IW (2000) *MacLeod's Clinical Examination*. 10th edn. Churchill
  Livingstone, London
Ogilvie C (1997) *Chamberlain's Symptoms and Signs in Clinical Medicine, an Introduction to
  Medical Diagnosis*. 12th edn. Butterworth Heinemann, London
Taylor D, Paton C, McConnell D, Kerwin R, eds (2003) *The Maudsley Prescribing Guidelines*.
  7th edn. Martin Dunitz, London
The Law Society (1995) *Assessment of Mental Capacity, Guidance for Doctors and Lawyers*.
  British Medical Association, London
World Health Organization (1992) *ICD-10: The ICD-10 Classification of Mental and
  Behavioural Disorders: Clinical Descriptions and Diagnostic Guidelines*. WHO, Geneva

Internet

The Department of Health, online at: http://www.doh.gov.uk
The Royal College of Psychiatrists, online at: http://www.rcpsych.ac.uk

Most internet search engines will bring up a list of 'MRCPsych Exam' preparation sites.

Reference

Sternbach H (1991) The serotonin syndrome. *Am J Psychiatry* **148**(6): 705–13

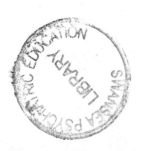